CALICO PUBLISHING

DEALING DAILY WITH DEMENTIA

Angela Caughey began writing in the mid-1980s, and is the author of four previous books. For more than 12 years she took care of her husband, who had dementia. She read widely around the subject, but found that none of the books included the practical hints for carers that she and her support group needed. She brings these together here for the benefit of all carers.

Other Health Books from Calico Publishing

*Positively Parkinson's: Symptoms & Diagnosis,
Research & Treatment, Advice & Support*
by Ann Andrews

*Chronic Fatigue Syndrome/M.E.: Symptoms,
Diagnosis, Management*
by Dr Rosamund Vallings MNZM, MB BS

Dying: A New Zealand Guide for the Journey
by Sue Wood and Peter Fox,
with Karen McMillan

www.calicopublishing.co.nz

Dealing Daily with Dementia

2000+ PRACTICAL HINTS & STRATEGIES FOR CARERS

Angela Caughey

calico

Calico Publishing Ltd
P O Box 29039
Greenwoods Corner
Auckland 1347
Phone and Fax: +64 9 6245674
www.calicopublishing.co.nz

© Angela Caughey 2013

ISBN 978-1-877429-07-1

A catalogue record for this book is available from the National Library of New Zealand

NEUROLOGICAL FOUNDATION OF NEW ZEALAND

Publication is generously assisted by the Neurological Foundation of New Zealand

This book is copyright. Apart from fair dealing for the purpose of private study, research, criticism or review, as permitted under the Copyright Act, no part may be reproduced by any process without the prior permission of the publisher.

The information included in this book is to be used as a guide only. The author, publisher and agents do not take responsibility for the application of this information.

Editor: Claire Gummer
Illustrations: Sally Hollis-McLeod
Cover design: Katy Yiakmis
Interior design: Julie McDermid
Typesetting: Punaromia Publications Ltd
Printed in China

*To Brian and his inspiring example of years
of uncomplaining courage*

If the drink that satisfied
    the son of Mary when he died
    has not the right smack for you
    leave it for a kindlier brew.

For my bitter verses are
    sponges steeped in vinegar
    useless to the happy-eyed
    but handy for the crucified.

R A K Mason

Contents

Foreword 9
Acknowledgements 11
Introduction 15

Part One   When It All Starts   21
1   Early Signs   23
2   The Doctor and the Diagnosis   29
3   Understanding Dementia   35
4   Dealing with the News   50
5   Legal and Money Matters   59

Part Two   Making Adjustments   67
6   Becoming a Carer   69
7   Dealing with Health Professionals   81
8   Adapting the Home Environment   90
9   Managing Difficult Behaviour   101
10   Wider Support and Self-care   110

Part Three   Balancing Acts   117
11   Independence and Safety   119
12   Feelings   127
13   Communication   140
14   Intimacy, Love and Sex   155

Part Four   Making Life Easier   167
15 Maintaining Health   169
16 Exercise   182
17 Entertainment   194
18 Holidays and Travel   210

Part Five   Practical Strategies for Managing   221
19 Eating and Drinking   223
20 Showering and Dressing   232
21 Toileting   244
22 Wandering   256
23 Hallucinations, Delusions and Delirium   262
24 Aggression   268

Part Six   The Later Stages   281
25 Choosing Full-time Care   283
26 Moving into Full-time Care   294
27 Final Days   310

Useful Resources   320
Select Bibliography   322
Index   327

Foreword

As we are belatedly becoming aware, dementia is a major health and social issue that will only become more significant as the population ages. Each person with dementia will have someone who is their main carer and many others will also be affected – from family, friends, neighbours, volunteers and health professionals to bus drivers, bank staff and passers-by. Governments and local councils and governing bodies are now beginning to consider the implications having of such large numbers of cognitively impaired people in our midst.

Unfortunately, there is no cure in sight, but this does not mean there is nothing to do. We can ensure that each person with dementia, their carers and family live as well as possible, despite the difficulties faced during the course of this relentlessly progressive condition. To do this we can learn much from the people who have trodden the caring path before us.

Angela Caughey is a carer writing a book for carers. She understands the life of caring for someone with dementia and the myriad challenges that are faced daily. Her book contains many practical strategies gleaned from her own journal and her support group of people in similar situations. Her suggestions are vividly (and often amusingly) illustrated with vignettes from her own and others' experiences. The book is chock-full of sensible and imaginative advice, yet still encourages people to find their own solutions.

The challenges to living well with dementia come not only from the condition itself or the changed skills of the person with dementia, but also from paid caregivers, professionals and the wider community. Angela rightly points out that people with dementia are still stigmatised, and often they and their caregivers become isolated and ignored. And, as she says here, it does not have to be like this. When dementia is diagnosed, people do not stop being themselves. It is hurtful if friends and family stay away because they are embarrassed and awkward, or think their absence won't be noticed. Stigma can lead to a delay in diagnosis and failure to access the voluntary and funded supports that are available. Nor should the diagnosis be kept from the person with dementia who needs to understand what is happening and plan for the future before it is too late.

Having information about how to manage always lessens the fear of the diagnosis. A brief look through the chapter titles will give you some idea of the breadth of topics covered; reading these chapters will give you an in-depth understanding of how to cope.

There will be times when the ongoing nature of care feels overwhelming and you are tempted to throw up your hands in hopelessness and helplessness. That is when you need a friend who understands, can laugh and weep with you and encourage you on the way. No one should be alone when caring for someone with any chronic health condition, and dementia is more challenging than most. This book encourages people to seek help from whoever can best provide it. Indeed the book itself could become one of your best companions along the way.

Dr Chris Perkins, MB ChB, FRANZCP
Specialist in old-age psychiatry

Acknowledgements

If this book helps others it is because of my co-carers' unique contributions. These give abundant testimony to their spirit and determination, and I am enormously grateful to them.

The following people have told their stories (anonymously, as requested) or lent their expertise and friendship in differing amounts in dozens of spheres. They will all know what they contributed and how much I owe them. I hope they are rewarded by the thought that their efforts may help people in future who are coping with dementia. My thanks to: Julie Agate, Sally Anderson, Rosie Ashby, Right Reverend Peter Atkins, Jean and Alex Baillie, Simon Barclay, Cilla Barkhuison, Roger and Bryan Bartley, Meg Bayley, Noel Bierre, Hilary Birch, Peter and Anne Blomfield, Kay Bodle, Sue Brewster, Glenys Bullivant, Mack Butts, Jenny and John Buxton, Ann and Iain Campbell, Judith Carr, Noel Cashmore, Bill and Shona Caughey, David and Elizabeth Caughey, Richard and Naomi Caughey, Chris Cole-Catley, Jenny and Martin Cole, Mavis Coleman, Jo Cory-Wright, Gillian Coulam, Ruskin Cranwell, Raewyn Davies, Sue Donaldson, David Dove, Richard Faull, Marilyn Flewett, Suzanne Frearson, Alan Gibb, Jonathan Gunson, Mike Hall, Ron Haydon, Deborah and Jo Heays, Margie Henderson, Jean Hook, Jim Horrocks, Irene Horton, Dône Hulley, Val Hyland, Wendy Innes, Pam Johnston, the Very Reverend Jo Kelly-Moore, June Kendrick, Jan Lawrence, Audrey Leaf, Cherry Long, Joan-Mary Longcroft, Annabelle Lord, Joy Lord, Jill Macindoe, Faye Macnicol, Melinda McCarthy, Donald McCulloch, Robyn McElroy, Kay McGarry, Roger McLean, Shirley Anne McNamara, Bruce Marler,

Anne Martin, Mission Bay Women's Bowling Club members, Colleen Montford, Geraldine Moore, Laurence Morton, Valerie Napier, Nanette Norris, Alison North, Chris Perkins, Jeanette Plunkett, Carol Pollock, Ann Proctor, Janet Robertson, Anton Roche, Tony and Phillip Sage, Laurie Smith, Barry Snow, Margaret Spencer, Isobel Stanton, Riri Stark, Heather Stivey, Russell Stone, Adele Taylor, Marie Taylor, Leone Venville, Heather Walker, Howard Waterfall, Janie Weir, Joan and Alastair Whitelaw, Delyse Whorwood, Barbara Wilson and Mary Rose Wilson.

Mention must be made of the people working in the caring field without whose help I should have floundered miserably: Dale and her staff at the Meadowbank Day Care, the owners and staff at Cromwell and Aranui Hospitals, the matron and staff at the Caughey Preston Hospital, the team at Auckland Health, home helpers Peggy, Maureen, Ann, Anil, Kei, Juliet and others, St Aidan's church vicars and office workers, the librarians at the Remuera branch of the Auckland library service, the managers and staff at Alzheimers Auckland and Alzheimers New Zealand, Hospice New Zealand, Max Ritchie, Jon Simcock and Sue Giddens and the team at the Neurological Foundation of New Zealand, Parkinson's Auckland and The Parkinsonism Society of New Zealand (Inc).

I am also humbled by and grateful to the people with dementia whose dozens of snippets of advice are sprinkled throughout the text. I can give them no individual recognition, but value their contributions for their wisdom and expressions of honest, poignant feelings.

As always, my family and their spouses and my grandchildren have been interested and supportive, and have given me space without letting me feel neglected; and I am also enormously grateful for the extensive and effective editing done by Claire Gummer, and the total friendship and support I received from her and my publisher, Linda Cassells. I enjoyed immensely working with them both and could not have had two more empathetic and capable people helping me on the way.

Permission was kindly given by the following to reproduce or draw from extracts in their publications: Alzheimers Auckland, 'Mind Matters', 2008 (in Chapter 17: Entertainment, 'Toolshed tasks'); Christine Boden,

Acknowledgements

Who Will I Be When I Die?, HarperCollins Religious, 1998 (in Chapter 3: Understanding Dementia, 'Early-onset dementia'); Jane Brotchie, *Caring for Someone with Dementia*, Age Concern Books, 2003 (in Chapter 4: Dealing with the News, 'Covering up'; and in Chapter 12: Feelings, 'Identifying your feelings' and 'Humour'); Lynne Bye, Liaison Officer for the Northern Division of the Pharmacy Guild (for the list in Chapter 15: Maintaining Health, 'When a medication is prescribed'); Brian McNaughton, 'God in Dementia', 'Alzheimer's News', June 2002 (in Chapter 12: Feelings, 'Spirituality'); Julia Millen, *Dilemma of Dementia*, Lansdowne Press, 1985 (in Chapter 7: Dealing with Health Professionals, 'Abilities and knowledge'; and Chapter 18: Holidays and Travel, 'What to tell your travel companion'); *New Zealand Listener*, 23 August 2008 (in Chapter 6: Becoming a Carer, 'Avoid contradiction'); *Penstrokes* magazine for the Carer's Code in Chapter 10: Wider Support and Self-care. My thanks also to the Hocken Library for permission to use R A K Mason's poem in the epigraph.

Introduction

So you find yourself caring for someone who has dementia? Welcome to the club. If you are doing this full time you may feel increasingly pushed and often extremely tired, but at times are surprised by a compensating sense of satisfaction. At least, that's what we found, the group of carers from whom the seeds for this book sprouted. We were women whose husbands had Lewy body dementia, and we belonged to a support group that met monthly for a café lunch.

The support organisation that had brought us together reckoned that we would be good for each other in the struggle ahead. And we were. Shyness with complete strangers evaporated quickly as we shared our inadequacies, difficulties and doubts. We began looking forward eagerly to our gatherings, to sitting round a table scattered with sandwiches, muffins and assorted drinks, confiding in each other.

Often we laughed out loud, with the other café patrons looking on in amusement, as we shared the hilarious situations our demented husbands got us into, or their odd hallucinations. At other times we were left speechless as we absorbed the implications of what we were hearing, and what might lie ahead. One of us might have had a particularly bad time since last we met, and the others would listen sympathetically, containing their own needs, while she unburdened herself. Sometimes we had already been through what she was describing. More often we had not; so we listened, noted, remembered, and when a similar situation developed in our own homes, we drew on these stories to avoid doing anything unwise and to respond in ways we had heard were successful.

The dementia books we were reading covered symptoms and medical aspects of the condition, but practical hints on how to cope with what we were facing were harder to come by. Our medical specialists acknowledged that they didn't really know enough to give advice about what carers have to deal with in their own homes. Someone in our group said we should publish all our strategies and suggestions in the Parkinson's magazine. But they grew beyond a magazine article. They grew into a book, the publication of which the specialists encouraged.

This book is the result of our pooling of ideas. It contains more than 2000 practical hints and strategies to help people who care for someone with this condition. Most of the content is written for people like us, caring for much loved (or not much loved!) spouses, partners, parents, or other relatives. But other people, who, perhaps, are being paid to care for those with dementia, may benefit from it too. Health professionals can gain more understanding of the day-to-day challenges presented by this widespread but diverse condition, and of practical ways to deal with them.

Encountering dementia

The number of people with dementia is increasing. Statistics have varied, but in 2012 the World Health Organization put it at 35 million worldwide, predicting that this figure would double by 2030 and more than triple by 2050. Research continues to uncover different causes for dementia symptoms, and finding ways to alleviate them. Such discoveries can make a difference, so long as several related goals of WHO are met. Those important goals include diagnosing dementia early, increasing support for carers and reducing the stigma of the disease.

Fifty years ago people never mentioned cancer; and 30 years ago depression was not something you would talk about. Now these conditions are discussed more freely, and we try to encourage rather than exclude the people who have them. Unfortunately, dementia still carries a stigma, but it is simply an organic disease, like emphysema or heart problems, and should be seen in a matter-of-fact way. If we can talk openly about it, then perhaps attitudes to the disease will be transformed. We have deliberately used the word dementia in the title of this book. The person you care for doesn't want to feel stigmatised, and although they feel their limitations very deeply, they want to be part of normal everyday life for as long as possible.

My first contact with dementia involved my godmother, Mrs A. As a child, I loved visiting her comfortable home and amazing garden. She was tall and slim, with a triangular, smiley face; large green eyes under wiry eyebrows; wavy, copper-grey hair; and a high-pitched laugh. She made me laugh too, while I looked in vain to see the 'green fingers' my mother had mentioned.

In my twenties I left my hometown. Visiting 10 years later, I went to see my godmother, now in care. Mrs A was almost unrecognisable: an ancient, white-haired, shrunken woman, strapped into a wheelchair, dribbling and mumbling indistinctly. I pulled up a chair and sat beside her. Her fingers restlessly pleated her nightgown, so that her legs and private parts became exposed. She took no notice of me.

Feeling inadequate, I told her my name. To my surprise her fingers stopped pleating, her nightdress fell down and her mumbles turned to words. I strained to hear. She was talking sense! She rattled on about the little Morris car she used to drive in the 1930s, her dead son's racing pigeons, how to make a sponge cake. I was amazed and comforted to find that she wasn't lost beyond the realms of reason. She was still Mrs A, and she was talking about matters that I recalled, even though her timeframe was astray.

That visit provided a valuable lesson: dementia means you have lost some (or lots) of your mental capacity, but you're still you.

Thirty years later I was again brought face to face with dementia, this time involving my managing-director husband. I cared for Brian at home for 12 years before his increasing dementia meant I could manage no longer. I chose one of his occasional lucid moments to tell him this, and he responded in his almost inaudible voice, 'If I go into permanent care I won't last more than five months.'

When he went into care, he deliberately stopped eating and started wasting away. After four weeks he choked on a drink, developed pneumonia a few days later, and died within 24 hours. He may have had severe dementia, but he was still as much in control of his life as he could be, still the managing director he had always been. He didn't want to go on living with the severe handicaps he carried. He just needed loving care – not to have his life protected and protracted by invasive medical expertise.

Various experiences of ours – mine and Brian's – are among those recorded in this book. Others come from many sources: our support group, people who have dementia, research reading, acquaintances with similar problems, and people who love a good joke – because laughter is one of the most valuable tonics for everyone concerned.

How to use this book

The stories and comments in these pages are crucial. They show the humanity of people with dementia, and of their carers. They are not included to tell you what to do, but to offer you choices to consider and weigh up and find out what works for you and the person you are taking care of. The same is true of the comprehensive range of practical hints presented. Overall, the aim is to make caring for a person with dementia much easier.

This was not planned as a book to sit down and read from start to finish – though you may choose to do that. Nor is it a medical text, though it may help you to work alongside, and assist, your doctors. It is a book made up of many basic details, and although some readers will think them trivial, others will find them useful. You too are facing a new experience – so fairly full, fundamental details will not go amiss.

Some people will go straight to Chapter 5: Legal and Money Matters, as it is vital to act on this information early. Others may respond immediately to the suggestion in Chapter 6: Becoming a Carer to keep a journal: this regular recording helped me to make sense of what was happening and to keep going with my care. Assistant carers or more distant family members may learn much from Chapter 1: Early Signs and Chapter 10: Wider Support and Self-care. For each reader, a different part of the book may resonate.

If you have limited time, or are already feeling stretched, you may find it best to use the contents in a self-directed, purposeful way. Look up key words in the index, as well as consulting the table of contents. Don't be surprised if you find that a single paragraph or small subsection offers several ways around a problem, or that you keep reading because you are led on by the ideas and practical tips you come across.

Even if you have read only a small part of a chapter, note the cross-references that crop up and check the 'Where to from here' section at the end of it, as frequently other pages will have complementary information. Use the subheadings within chapters, too, to help you find more material that's relevant to you.

The way ahead

You will have some failures. They are normal and there is no need to be ashamed of them. We can learn from our failures, adapt and go forward better equipped as a result, and with more understanding. Also, any carer or person with dementia who continues to anguish – over unfashionable clothing, stains on carpets, spilt food, jumbled messages or repetitive behaviour – is going to be unhappy. They will constantly fight the inevitable. So be a normal, fallible, warm human being.

Choose the course of action you think is best, laugh, accept your mistakes, and try not to be a die-hard perfectionist. The carers of people with dementia who deal most honestly, uncomplainingly and willingly with their lot may find surprising times of consolation and contentment – despite many moments of thinking 'Why did this have to happen to me?' or 'How long will this go on?', and the accompanying feelings of frustration, impatience or exhaustion.

There is no 'proper' way to be a carer. Both you and the person you are looking after are unique personalities. You need to create your own workable partnership to manage the difficulties ahead. Living with dementia is going to be as straightforward as your attitudes and partnership make it.

PART ONE

When It All Starts

Chapter 1

Early Signs

The first noticeable thing about the person you'd known for a long time may have been that they appeared out of sorts, or their behaviour was out of character. They could even seem to ignore you or dislike you – a change that, if exhibited by your spouse, could lead you to consider separation or divorce.

It would be natural to wonder whether this grumpiness was just part of the ageing process. There may be nothing specific you could report to your doctor, and you'd hesitate to mention anything to the person you were worrying about. So you carried on, day by day finding life was becoming more and more difficult and demanding. These are common situations, although your story is unique and symptoms vary with the person involved.

Losing things, forgetfulness

Early signs of dementia can include losing things, though this is not an unusual experience for people in middle age and beyond. But there is a difference between normal memory loss and early dementia.

> Bernard and Georgia fulfilled a lifetime dream when he retired from his manufacturing business: they went to live near a golf course.
> But, within a year, Bernard was often confused.
> Georgia found his 'important papers' in the pantry. 'How on earth did they get there?' he asked before she could ask him the same question. 'I've no idea,' she replied, feeling defensive. The next week his 'lost' wallet turned up in the fridge, and his

reading glasses were found under a bush eight weeks after he couldn't find them, by which time they had been replaced.

When Bernard drove her to the supermarket to buy the week's supplies soon after, Georgia had to face reality. When she came out, laden with plastic bags, there was no sign of him or the car. After waiting half an hour with mounting suspicions she found a public phone box and rang their neighbour. 'Hi, Bill, is there any sign of life at our place?'

'Sure is, Georgia,' he said cheerfully. 'All the lights are on and I can see Bernard comfortably settled with the paper and a glass of wine. Why do you ask? Where are you?'

Of course, forgetfulness does not always equate to dementia. Carers, who are understandably sensitive to signs of cognitive decline, can start believing that they, too, are showing symptoms as they find themselves forgetting names and losing words in the middle of sentences. The comparisons below show what is considered to be normal memory loss and what is not.

Normal and abnormal memory loss

NORMAL MEMORY LOSS	NOT SO NORMAL
Forgetting where you left your cheque book	Forgetting which bank you use
Repeating a story to friend or spouse	Repeating a story over and over on the same day to the same person
Forgetting what you had for breakfast yesterday	Forgetting what you had for breakfast 15 minutes ago
Using calendars and lists to remind you to do certain things	Forgetting to use calendars and lists and not understanding the use of either of these
Being disoriented for a moment waking up in a strange motel room while travelling	Getting lost in your own home where you have lived for several years
Sometimes forgetting where you parked the car	Forgetting that you drove to the shops or that you have a car
Forgetting the details of a holiday 10 years ago	Forgetting that you went for a trip last week
Worrying that you have memory problems	Becoming unaware and uncaring that you have memory loss

Hallucinating, having delusions

For Alison and her competent, managing-director husband, the first suggestion anything was awry came when they were playing golf together.

One short, par three hole looked easy – just a simple 8 iron from an elevated tee over a stream and on to the green – but both Bruce and Alison put their balls into that water. They pulled their golf trundlers down to the hazard. The stream was running fast and deep so there was no chance of finding balls there. Alison groped in her bag for a replacement, pulled out a club, dropped the ball on to the grass, addressed it and chipped it safely over the water towards the flag.

She turned to see Bruce facing the green, holding his right arm and fist straight out to the side. He opened his hand, but no ball dropped. Nevertheless, he chose a club, addressed the non-existent ball, played a make-believe chip shot, put his club back into his bag, took the handle of his trundler and walked on to park it by the green. Slightly bemused, his wife followed.

'Where's my ball?' Bruce asked, as Alison approached to make her first putt. 'You didn't play a ball,' she answered. 'You looked as if you were going to drop one, but there was nothing in your hand.' They looked at each other. Nothing more was said just then; they played out the round. That was her introduction to Lewy body dementia (LBD) and the beginning of Bruce's journey.

Disorientation, aggression

The golf course experience with Bruce was baffling, but in itself posed no real problem. But sometimes the initial signs of early-onset dementia can be downright dangerous.

When his mother and aunt were killed in a car crash Jeffrey, the oldest son in his early fifties, took responsibility for handling the funeral arrangements. He did not cope well. He refused to talk about the subject, became withdrawn and, driving home from the funeral, caused a 10 to 12 car pile-up by stopping suddenly. He had no idea why he had braked.

During the next four years he increasingly talked in his sleep and thrashed about in the bed he shared with Janine, his wife, often punching her with what seemed to be well-aimed blows, although apparently still unconscious.

Sometime later he confessed to her that twice, when he had gone away on business, he had not known what to do when he arrived. Janine insisted he tell his doctor, an old family friend, who said Jeffrey was depressed and referred him to a stress counsellor. This man simply said his symptoms were typical of late fifties, tired, working males, and Jeffrey refused to go back to him.

Janine felt like a battered wife. Ashamed, she would not stay at a hotel after their son's wedding in case the family became aware of Jeffrey's night-time violence. She was increasingly disturbed by this, by his not taking responsibility for his deteriorating health, with his lack of interest in her and her activities, and by health professionals who said there was nothing wrong with him. She began to consider leaving him.

On a solo trip to Melbourne, Jeffrey would not go out by himself, did not even visit the Melbourne Cricket Ground (a lifelong ambition), and generally lacked confidence. Hearing of this, Janine regretted not going with him, as it was clear there was some pathological reason for his behaviour.

In this case, it took years before a medical professional mentioned dementia of any kind (Jeffrey had Lewy body dementia). Unfortunately this experience echoes that of other families where other disturbing symptoms have become evident.

Confusion, reduced ability to care for oneself

Another scenario for many is where, after the death of a spouse who has been covering up, forgetfulness and confusion in the surviving partner become increasingly obvious. They can become a danger to themselves, if not to anyone else.

Francie and her husband, Joseph, were a devoted, close couple in old age. They moved together to an apartment in a retirement village as she began to show signs of 'cognitive decline', but when Joseph died six months later, Francie became lost, irritable and very confused without him. Her son did his best to monitor her financial dealings but, despite his best efforts, she (who had been a high-powered, competent businesswoman) got into dreadful tangles. Sorting these out was made more difficult because she insisted she did not want or need any help. Her other adult children's responses varied from acceptance to denial of the ever-increasing signs of dementia, and her doctor (a specialist geriatrician) didn't help: he said that, although she was exhibiting 'age-related forgetfulness', he saw no cause for alarm.

The management of the retirement village was concerned about her deterioration, however, and the family arranged for an afternoon caregiver (telling Francie that this woman was lonely and needed company) but very soon the caregiver reported Francie's disasters in the kitchen and said she didn't think Francie should ever be left on her own. When the village's management ultimately said Francie would have to leave, her three daughters took her on a three-week cruise. During this time she was such a disorientated total liability that everyone realised – even the doubters – that her deterioration was more than the ageing process.

After returning home and three weeks 'under observation' in hospital, she was diagnosed with Alzheimer's disease and finally went into a secure dementia facility – completely dependent on the very caring staff. The family was amazed that it took so long for her to be diagnosed, yet suspected that, given her independent (bordering on stubborn) nature, it would have caused her huge distress to have been moved earlier against her wishes.

In most of the cases above, the people who were developing dementia were unaware of others' concerns and continued their lives normally for quite a while, in spite of what was creeping up on them.

It is worth encouraging your friends to absorb information about dementia as part of their general or 'life' knowledge, and to seek help early if their suspicions are raised.

Where to from here

+ Chapter 2: The Doctor and the Diagnosis
+ Chapter 3: Understanding Dementia
+ Chapter 4: Dealing with the News
+ Chapter 5: Legal and Money Matters
+ Chapter 7: Dealing with Health Professionals
+ Chapter 9: Managing Difficult Behaviour
+ Chapter 23: Hallucinations, Delusions and Delirium
+ Chapter 24: Aggression

Chapter 2

The Doctor and the Diagnosis

Ideal ways to reach a diagnosis

You, and the person you are worried about, decide to visit the family doctor when you have seen and experienced enough to feel that the memory loss and/or other symptoms may be more than 'a one-off' – but before life has become a struggle. You go together: two heads are better than one.

Your doctor listens carefully, does a complete physical examination and takes a detailed medical history. They order tests – physical (blood and urine) as well as mental (memory and skills). They also assess mood and emotions. Any more in-depth investigation after that may involve X-rays or scans, spinal fluid sampling or an EEG (testing electrical activity in the brain). The person may also see a specialist, or a clinical psychologist who does cognitive tests.

Dementia may not be the first word on your doctor's lips. One simple test won't reveal it, and anyway dementia is a diagnosis of exclusion: a conclusion that doctors can only reach after checking for (and eliminating) other possibilities such as stress or depression, which can also create memory problems. So if you are sent to a psychiatrist, rather than a neurologist or a geriatrician, this may be to rule out another condition.

If the problem is dementia, it is in everybody's interests to have this diagnosed as soon – and as accurately – as possible. Internationally, clinical criteria exist to help doctors do this. These include the NICE Guideline on Dementia (UK) and the Diagnostic Guidelines for Alzheimer's Disease (US). The latter were updated in 2011 in line with research advances.

Will it get better?

Dementia itself is irreversible, but on occasion dementia-like symptoms may be reversible – when caused by drugs, alcohol, imbalances of hormones or vitamins, or depression, rather than organic brain disease.

It is important to get checked out if there are sudden changes, rather than assume these are part of getting old or a worsening of existing dementia. Treatments can reduce or slow down the effects of some irreversible forms of dementia – another reason to press on with investigating and seeking a specific diagnosis.

See also Chapter 23: Hallucinations, Delusions and Delirium, 'Delirium'.

Down the track

Whether or not dementia is diagnosed, on first seeing a specialist your charge may take a mini mental status examination (MMSE) or the newer Addenbrooke's cognitive examination – revised (ACE–R). These help show where, and how much, the brain may be damaged.

When dementia is an accepted diagnosis, the mental tests occur regularly, with the latest and previous results compared. This allows the specialist to estimate the rate of deterioration. If there is a marked downturn, they may gloss over the score to maintain a positive approach. As time goes by, moreover, some people with dementia resist these tests – they can remember finding them difficult.

Sometimes a doctor will ask for a CT scan or other tests, if they notice changes in the MMSE results. Don't feel concerned if another test is suggested. We are lucky that these processes are available.

Questions to ask when the diagnosis is dementia

When dementia is diagnosed, discuss it fully with the doctor or specialist who has told you and take notes. Initial queries could include:
- How does this dementia usually develop?
- What other symptoms may appear?
- What treatments are available?
- What support services are available?

Again, it is preferable for both the patient and their support person to be there. (See Chapter 7: Dealing with Health Professionals.)

Common experiences during diagnosis

It can take years to get a dementia diagnosis, and surveys around the world have found that the condition is woefully underdiagnosed. You would have been concerned about the decreasing abilities of someone in your life, but have probably – understandably – delayed seeking medical advice.

When you finally went to the doctor, you all needed to work through the possibilities in a methodical way. Many family doctors feel ill-equipped to diagnose and manage dementia: in 2007 a UK report found that less than one-third felt they had the training they needed for this. Your doctor may have felt uncomfortable – or perceived that you were – given the stigma of dementia, and so handled it badly, or they may have oversimplified the medical description to avoid using the words 'senile dementia'.

You may have felt your doctor simply waffled before referring you on, and when you finally secured an appointment with a specialist, they too may have handled you with kid gloves.

> Well before he retired, Alan was having difficulty remembering business orders, and was commenting on his declining ability to read and understand.
>
> Two years after he stopped working, his driving was erratic and one foot dragged slightly when he walked. His family and Judy, his wife, wanted to know whether he might have a brain tumour or had a mini-stroke and wondered how to explain the hallucinations and changes in his mental functioning.
>
> Alan finally agreed to talk to his doctor about these issues after two more years. His doctor sent him to a neurologist, who diagnosed Parkinson's but, in a private report that only the doctor saw, also noted 'significant dementia'. Alan was shell-shocked by the diagnosis. Judy was distressed, too, though pleased to have, at last, an explanation and treatment for Alan's symptoms. The family doctor never mentioned dementia to either of them.

A year later, still perplexed, the couple sought another opinion – from a gerontologist. He agreed that Alan had Parkinson's, but added Alzheimer's to the diagnosis, naming dementia officially for the first time. Later still, eight years after the original symptoms, Alan was told by the support person from the national Parkinson's organisation that he had Lewy body dementia.

When the doctor won't say it's dementia

The experience above is not an isolated one. Sometimes medical professionals do not tell patients they have dementia, and carers are kept in the dark, with some reporting that no doctor ever mentioned 'dementia' to their face.

A retired surgeon, Keith, asked his daughter, before she went overseas, whether she noticed any changes in her mother. She replied noncommittally – but on returning five years later she did notice obvious changes, and how difficult her father's life had become. He was slaving away, caring for his wife, but never mentioning dementia.

Their family doctor appeared to see the surgeon as his senior and deferred to him, while the surgeon did not want to demean his wife or question their doctor's treatment. The wife was not finally diagnosed with Alzheimer's until another four years had passed. It was a relief for everyone, but the family felt the diagnosis should have been made much earlier.

According to Chris Perkins, a specialist in old-age psychiatry, most doctors who avoid telling patients or their carers of a dementia diagnosis do so in the belief – generally a mistaken one – that their patients don't want to know.

'I wish I had known all about what to expect,' said Iris. She had been in constant uncertainty during three years of looking after her husband, Roger, because they had never been given the dementia diagnosis. 'Our doctor thought that, if he told us what might happen, we would have spent all our time worrying about it or imagining it was about to hit us. But it would've been like travelling the main rail trunk line: you're on the train, you don't know what stations you are going to stop at, but you know their names as you pass by!'

Other carers and patients involved in this book have certainly found it helpful to be told the diagnosis. Knowing about the dementia helped them to start adapting their lives to cope positively with this 'new' condition.

> Alex did not know how much to tell his wife, who was in the early stages of dementia, but she knew him well enough to feel his indecision and told him they were in this thing together and never to hold back.

Although they have dementia, your charge is still able to understand, is the same person they were yesterday, and needs to be treated normally – just as though they have their full faculties.

Getting a second opinion

If you get no diagnosis at all, or if your experience doesn't match the diagnosis you do receive, you can seek a second opinion – or a third, or fourth – from another health professional who is qualified to give it.

> Janine, nearly at the end of her tether with Jeffrey, went to the medical school's library to do some research for herself. She read enough to decide that Jeffrey had Parkinson's disease and probably also Lewy body dementia – but she didn't have enough confidence to challenge his doctor, the geriatrician or the neurologist.
>
> After three more stressful years, Janine could take no more. She made an appointment for her husband with a different neurologist who, as soon as Jeffrey came into his consulting room, knew from his walk that he had Parkinson's. No other doctor had mentioned this in almost 10 years. The dementia diagnosis came soon after.

Where to from here
✦ Chapter 3: Understanding Dementia
✦ Chapter 4: Dealing with the News
✦ Chapter 5: Legal and Money Matters

- Chapter 7: Dealing with Health Professionals, especially 'Seeing a specialist'
- Chapter 6: Becoming a Carer
- Chapter 8: Adapting the Home Environment
- Chapter 10: Wider Support and Self-care
- Chapter 12: Feelings
- Chapter 15: Maintaining Health

Chapter 3

Understanding Dementia

More than a century after scientists began making important discoveries about dementia, much more research is needed to reveal its remaining secrets. In essence, 'dementia' describes how organic diseases affect brain cells, impairing a person's thinking, remembering and reasoning. It is not what most people would classify as a mental illness, but can show similar changes in mood, behaviour and even personality.

What goes on in the head of someone with dementia?

Imagine that schoolchildren in a class have agreed not to speak to or touch each other for a whole lesson. Suddenly, several children rush in late with exciting news. They write the news down, fold the paper into darts and throw these to others in the classroom. Their classmates catch the darts, read the news avidly, refold the darts and throw them on to others. Imagine that some of the darts are caught, but others aren't; they fall to the floor and form untidy heaps. The news does not get read or passed round to everyone and, as the children rush out at the end of the period, the heaps are trampled underfoot. Some children are confused about what exactly the exciting news was and what they were meant to do about it, but the darts are now unreadable scraps.

Similar confusion occurs in someone affected by dementia. People with the condition have described the results themselves:

> Every few months I sense that another piece of me is missing. I only think half thoughts. Some day I may never think again – maybe

not know who I am. We all expect to die some day, but whoever expected to lose themselves first?

♦

I am now living in what seems like a foreign place where I am lost, and the people I once knew are so different that I no longer recognise them.

♦

You are walking or sitting in a strange place, you don't know where you are and you feel quite sure that this is not where you should be. It isn't your home. Suddenly a stranger comes up to you, grabs your arm and tries to get you to do something out of the blue. You lash out in defence.

♦

It is like living in a place with a lot of strange people and you wish you might live somewhere on your own, not in this sort of place, where most of the people seem either quite mad or awfully dull. You vaguely remember that once you had another sort of life.

The complexity of the brain

The confusion that dementia creates in people is hardly surprising, as the human brain is like an unbelievably complicated computer. It has two hemispheres, each divided into four main lobes that specialise in different functions – problem-solving, visual recognition, behaviour and emotion, and so on. The brain's billions of cells form a motherboard which controls our whole body.

Normally, brain cells continually receive electrical impulse messages, like emails, from all over the body, via the spinal cord and cranial nerves. These messages are prompts for making decisions (What movement shall I make? What do I think about that?), decisions of which we are often unaware.

Each cell receives its message from an adjoining cell's terminal branches via the tips of its dendrites, which are finger-like extensions of the cell body. The cell takes the message to its cell body: its control centre. Here it integrates the message, then passes its judgement along to the

Understanding Dementia 37

Functions of different areas of the brain

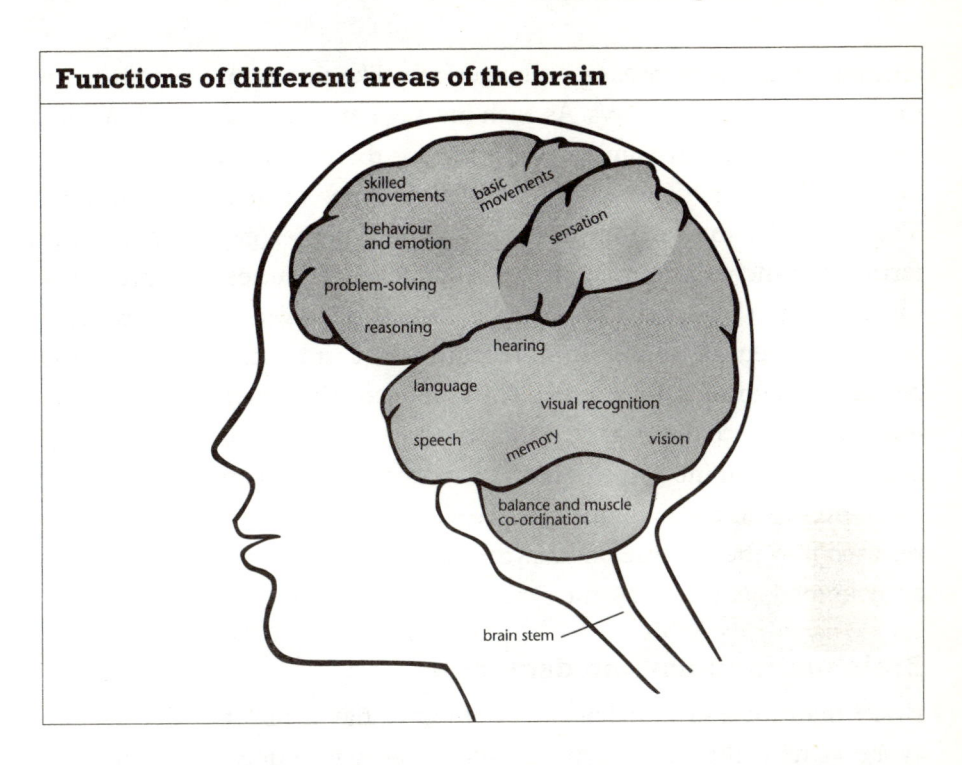

- skilled movements
- basic movements
- behaviour and emotion
- sensation
- problem-solving
- reasoning
- hearing
- language
- visual recognition
- speech
- memory
- vision
- balance and muscle co-ordination
- brain stem

Brain cells transmitting message

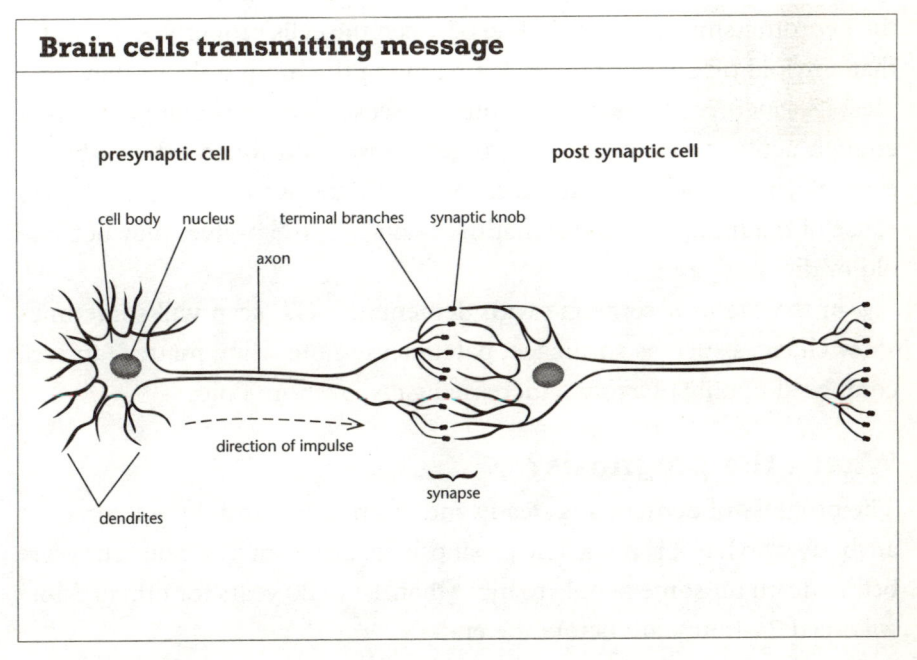

presynaptic cell

post synaptic cell

- cell body
- nucleus
- terminal branches
- synaptic knob
- axon
- direction of impulse
- synapse
- dendrites

terminal branches of its axon – a longer, arm-like extension – to transfer to the next cell's dendrite tip/s. As each message impulse reaches the axon's terminal branches, it stimulates the release there of a chemical called a neurotransmitter. (There are 15 different types of neurotransmitter.) This takes the message impulse across the synapse (gap) between the terminal branches and the next cell's dendrites. That next cell processes the message and passes it on along its axon in the same way, the process being repeated an almost infinite number of times as the message is passed like lightning from one cell to the next. Each cell contributes its own suggestion to the final decision on what action to take. In Lewy body dementia, dopamine is the neurotransmitter that is affected.

One of the main neurotransmitters is acetylcholine. After this is released into the synapse, an enzyme called acetylcholinesterase clears it away immediately, leaving the synapse ready for more messages.

Brain malfunction and dementia

Brain malfunction that leads to dementia has a number of possible causes. One is that the enzyme acetylcholinesterase does not clear away the neurotransmitter acetylcholine between the cells properly. A second is that amyloid plaques or tangles form among the brain cells, so they send messages incorrectly, as in Alzheimer's disease. A third is that people lack enough active neurotransmitter to get messages through efficiently; for example, insufficient dopamine can lead to Parkinson's disease. A fourth cause of brain malfunction is that the brain cells themselves may become old or diseased, and die.

In the brain of someone with dementia, a CT scan will sometimes show changes such as shrinkage, patchiness in the white matter (an area composed mainly of axons), increased gaps, or more fluid.

What's the prognosis?

The progress of dementia is steady and often rapid, and the outcome for anybody who has it is poor. The prognosis ranges from less than four years before death for some people to more than 10 to 20 years for others. Most will need 24-hour care before the end.

Forms of dementia

Dozens of different conditions are categorised as dementia. The form a person develops depends not only on which lobe of the brain is affected, but also which part of the lobe – and some people have more than one form of dementia. Also, some diagnoses can only be conclusively made on autopsy, though generally enough signs are evident earlier for a doctor to give an informed judgement.

Every individual with dementia lives with an unwanted cocktail of symptoms from the same long list of possibilities. One result of recent and ongoing study is the blurring of dementia classifications. In a sense, too, the important thing is not 'naming' your dementia but continuing to give the person affected the same respect and attention as you would any friend.

However, names can still be useful, and since each identified form of dementia has slightly different symptoms, it can help to know which of these may develop in the person you are caring for. Several of the better-known dementias are described below.

Alzheimer's disease

Alzheimer's disease (AD) is the most common form of dementia in the West, accounting for probably 60 per cent of cases. Approximately twice as many women as men develop it. Some rare forms of the disease are inherited, and early-onset Alzheimer's occurs infrequently.

Alzheimer's leads to 'death by small steps' for a brain addled by tangles and plaques. Symptoms may progress quite quickly, or may be of minor importance beside competing health problems like cancer or other diseases which kill the person before AD runs its course. An Alzheimer's diagnosis can only be confirmed by autopsy, although researchers are seeking ways to confirm it earlier.

In a person still living normally, loss of words and short-term memory are among the first indications of AD, with vocabulary and talking ability gradually deteriorating.

> Evelyn, an intelligent, well-groomed perfectionist, turned to her
> daughter one day and said, 'Oh, bother, look at all this – ah, what's-

its-name – this yellow sticky stuff on my shoe.' She had lost the word 'clay'.

Eight years on, a neighbour showed Evelyn a pattern book for the children's toys she was knitting. Evelyn browsed through some of the illustrations, and then commented, 'What a lot of lovely, colourful grandchildren you have!'

When she moved into full-time care several years later, Evelyn conversed only with her constantly cuddled best friend – her teddy bear.

Despite their confusion, people with AD will still act independently as well as make and respond to jokes.

Duncan, who had been caring for his wife Evelyn for several years, would find half-finished glasses of gin in surprising places. He tried hiding the gin bottle in an upstairs top cupboard – but Evelyn found it. She didn't pour herself a gin, but decorated the bottle with pieces of gift ribbon, carefully put it back and, next time her daughter came to visit, she led her upstairs. 'Come and look at this,' she giggled. 'Dad hid the gin bottle from me but I found it – and I'm just letting him know with the ribbon effect!'

They feel emotions and will express and act on them:

A specialist trying to determine how far dementia had advanced in his patient subjected her insensitively to a battery of questions and commands. She gave no cooperation, ignored him for a while and then asked to lie down. When she had lain down on the first aid bed in another room, she snorted to her carer, 'Who does he think he is, that man? He's so bossy and self-important. Now that I've got away from him, tell me when he goes and I'll get up again.'

People with Alzheimer's are usually capable of responding to music, including songs such as hymns, and of interacting with others. They also retain other everyday abilities such as repeating deeply learned words, movements and gestures, expressing ideas, telling stories and responding appropriately to most situations.

An Alzheimer's brain eventually forgets how to run the body; how, for example, to chew and swallow (see Chapter 19: Eating and Drinking,

'Help with swallowing'). Coma and death eventually come between four and 20 years after diagnosis.

Vascular dementia

This is the most prevalent dementia among Asians, but the second most common type in the rest of the world. It is caused by a stroke, or multiple strokes. In these, blood flow to the brain is blocked by a clot or thickening of the walls of small arteries, or lost when an artery bursts, and the blood vessels and cells fed by that blood are deprived of oxygen and die.

After-effects of a stroke are mainly physical impairment of movement and speech: the mind knows what it wants to say, but the tongue won't produce the words. It is easy to think this is because of dementia, but it isn't. That comes later after more strokes. These impairments, plus dizziness, weakness and increasing confusion, indicate that vascular dementia is developing.

Unlike Alzheimer's, vascular dementia can sometimes be prevented by treating high blood pressure (and for warning signs, see Chapter 15: Maintaining Health, 'Watching out for strokes'). The symptoms of vascular dementia are very similar to those for Alzheimer's and some people have both – an example of mixed dementia.

Major features are unpredictable behaviour and changeable emotions such as weeping, anger, aggression, crying or laughing inappropriately. Someone with vascular dementia can lose control over basic reactions, or their responses may not reflect what they are really feeling. If they rant and swear this may be their only way to express frustration given their new difficulty in finding the right words.

> Stewart, a fit, squash-playing bloke, had a stroke at 43 and was unconscious for several days. Tracey, his wife, was in his room with a group of nurses when he opened his eyes. He struggled to sit up and let loose a string of the foulest language Tracey had ever heard. He had certainly never used those words in front of her before, and she didn't know he even knew them. But the nurses all cheered him on, saying 'Oh good, good, good, Mr Finlay, congratulations, you're talking well. Keep it up!'

When Stewart finally came home from hospital, swearing was still his main form of conversation and, despite Tracey's best efforts, he never did learn to speak clearly again, although sometimes he was able to write down a key word to help get his meaning across. He took his frustrations out with occasional physical violence, and running in every available marathon.

With or without dementia, a stroke may bring clumsiness or an altered sensation in the limbs or face. The person can, as with other forms of dementia, be apathetic, depressed, and have difficulty concentrating due to damage in parts of the brain which control enthusiasm, energy and motivation. They may also lose their sense of time and, sporadically, short-term memory.

Martha had had several strokes and TIAs [transient ischaemic attacks: small strokes] and wobbled along very slowly with her walker. After another attack her family took her to a lakeside cabin as a birthday treat and, during four quiet days there, she often expressed thanks. Then they returned her home, where all the medical and toilet equipment she would now need had been installed while she was away.

An old friend called the day after her return and asked how the holiday had gone. 'What holiday?' Martha asked. 'I don't know what you're talking about.'

Some abilities may be little altered, since vascular dementia affects the brain in a patchy way. Also, in some areas where their abilities deteriorate, they may develop compensating behaviours. For instance, if they lose their ability to understand speech, they may still understand by reading or looking at pictures, because these skills are found in another lobe of the brain which may be less affected.

They may remain physically healthy and eat well. Personality remains relatively intact, except in rare cases, and people with vascular dementia are more aware of their disability than are those with Alzheimer's. However, if they were very independent before their stroke, they may feel they have lost control over their own lives and may attempt activities that are unrealistic and beyond their abilities.

Other neurological effects of strokes

A stroke on one side of your brain affects control of movements on the opposite side of the body. If you find you can't wiggle your right thumb, it is because the left side of your brain can't give it instructions, and vice versa.

Left hemisphere damage

If a stroke has affected the brain's left side, your charge may have trouble with thinking logically and using factual material in a rational way. Processing information one step at a time may be difficult. Likewise, someone who was previously mathematically adept may struggle to work with numbers and symbols, or to analyse advanced mathematical problems.

Damage to the brain's left side also affects speech, reading and writing, remembering acts, recalling names or dates, and spelling. Musical talent may remain, however, together with the ability to use words correctly when singing.

> Pamela had a glorious singing voice. After a debilitating stroke she rallied, but then had more TIAs and dementia became established. She remained unaware of her condition, believing things were going along normally: in fact her husband was giving her 24-hour care.
>
> At the lunch party he arranged for her seventy-fifth birthday, Pamela greeted everyone with her usual outgoing, friendly warmth – and tumbling, senseless words. She was a gracious hostess but unable to communicate verbally, until the sing-song. Then her still-true voice soared above everyone else's, her words correct and audible.

Right hemisphere damage

If a stroke has damaged the brain's right side, your charge may have trouble learning through images and pictures, or recognising faces. Empathy and understanding can deteriorate, as can the ability to evaluate a whole problem at once. Doing jigsaws and finding their way around the house may be difficult. Ability to understand metaphors and imagery is lost too:

if somebody says, 'He's really on my back', the damaged right brain will take it literally. The stroke-affected person loses the ability to make up stories, speculate, imagine or wonder 'What if…?'

This kind of stroke reduces innate musical talent and the ability to respond to music, although if the person studied music when young, their left hemisphere will have absorbed music as well. It also affects drawing, painting and sculpting; expression of feelings; making love; worship, prayer and mysticism.

Epilepsy

It is not unusual for stroke victims to develop epilepsy in later years. For one couple whose needs had previously fallen under the radar of the health system, this brought an unexpected side-effect:

> Tracey spent the next 30 years caring for Stewart at home after his stroke and subsequent dementia and epilepsy. His marathon running eventually wore out his hips. Someone forgot to give him his epilepsy medication while he was in hospital for a hip replacement, and he had a major epileptic seizure and fell out of bed. For the first time, he was assigned a case manager, had a thorough assessment and went immediately into full-time care.

Lewy body dementia

Lewy body dementia (LBD) began to be diagnosed in the mid-1990s and is still sometimes missed by doctors. It may, however, be responsible for about 15 per cent of dementias. Your charge may initially have been told they had Alzheimer's or Parkinson's, because some of their symptoms are similar, and indeed LBD can coexist with them and other dementias.

The Lewy bodies (abnormal collections of protein in the brain) can cause degeneration and death of brain cells as well as disrupt neurotransmitters' work. They can also be present in Parkinson's, although in a different part of the brain.

The Parkinson-like symptoms that people with LBD can develop include stiffness and/or trembling, slow and shuffling gait with short steps, and an increasing tendency to break into a run and then fall.

> Ann took Reg's hand as they climbed up the grassy slope to the museum. He had been diagnosed with LBD only two weeks previously and she felt very protective. But she now felt helpless as his stooped Parkinson's-like walk became more and more pronounced and turned into a wobbly run. His nose got closer and closer to the slope and he finally collapsed onto the grass.
>
> She had been pulling his hand to hold him up, but she only managed to strain her shoulder. She learned later to stop them both walking when she noticed Reg's steps getting shorter and quicker.

Lewy bodies are only identifiable under autopsy, so diagnosis of LBD is difficult. It is essential, though, because drugs prescribed sometimes for Parkinson's or other dementias can have unpleasant effects on people with LBD, while acetylcholinesterase inhibitors (AChEIs) can be more effective in LBD than in Alzheimer's. (See Chapter 15: Maintaining Health, 'Cautionary notes'.) A doctor can narrow the diagnosis to LBD by noting the adverse effects of these drugs along with such symptoms as hallucinations and falls.

This form of dementia has plateaus, and people who have it deteriorate in steps, rather than declining steadily. At times, all the way through, the person you are caring for may seem like their old self, although lucidity can vary from hour to hour, even minute to minute. Over time they may show difficulty with short-term memory, judgement and putting words together. Reading, writing, reasoning and calculating skills may decline, and with these changes the ability to gauge space and distance can also decrease; for instance, a previously adept host may continue 'filling' a guest's glass even as it overflows.

As with Parkinson's, the person's face may become increasingly expressionless, and they may feel depression and anxiety. Movements are slower and their voice may be hard to hear.

They may hallucinate – visually at first, later involving touch and smell (see Chapter 23: Hallucinations, Delusions and Delirium). Abnormal beliefs or delusions are features in LBD. Sleep disorders relating to rapid eye movement (REM) have often been apparent for years previously, and the person may have vivid dreams, when they may call or strike out in their sleep (see Chapter 1: Early Signs, 'Disorientation, aggression').

Other expressions of LBD include fainting, falls or unexplained turns, dizziness on standing, and toileting accidents.

Parkinson's disease dementia

Not everyone who develops Parkinson's goes on to develop dementia. However, if dementia appears in your charge more than a year after a Parkinson's diagnosis, it generally follows the path of Parkinson's disease dementia (PDD). If dementia appears within the year, the original diagnosis should be reconsidered: the condition may in fact have been LBD, and this could affect the medications being used.

The most common initial PDD symptoms include stiffness or tremors, loss of facial expression, loss of memory and reasoning ability, not being able to carry out normal everyday tasks, loss of emotional control.

> Tom had always said, 'If you are not prepared, be prepared to fail,' yet half an hour before their son's wedding he had not realised that his shirt button was too tight to do up, and had mislaid his speech.
>
> Two or more years later, after his wife had been alarmed by lots of disquieting events, Tom collapsed at a conference. Parkinson's and its accompanying dementia were diagnosed.
>
> They kept this secret for a while; but, when they finally opened up, they realised friends had suspected something was wrong.
>
> Some rallied around, others didn't.

Less common effects of PDD arising from medications such as ropinirole (available as Requip) include atypical gambling, shoplifting and other behaviour. It is easy to ignore a person affected by Parkinson's disease if they have an expressionless face – those around them should make an effort to include them.

Fronto-temporal dementias

Fronto-temporal dementia (FTD) involves damage to the brain's frontal and temporal lobes. Its occurrence is significant among younger people, especially ages 40–60.

One of the three main types of FTD affects personality and behaviour; another attacks language and speaking skills; and a third has its effect on movement. Pick's disease is one of a number of rare forms of FTD. Like Lewy body dementia, it involves abnormal collections of protein (in this instance 'Pick bodies') in the brain, and can only be conclusively diagnosed on autopsy.

Fronto-temporal dementias in general are extremely difficult to diagnose accurately. The person can have an extraordinary range of symptoms that follow no fixed pattern and can change over time. Sometimes these are misdiagnosed initially as bipolar disorder, schizophrenia, deep depression or Alzheimer's.

The person affected may lack insight, or may be aware of their peculiar behaviours yet be unable to stop them. They may seem easily distracted, unable to plan, and lacking in financial judgement.

> 'I tried to dig a drain with the ride-on mower,' Charles began, adding that it seemed a perfectly normal thing to do. His wife reported, 'He would put the wrong petrol in the car and hoe up flowers I had planted. Some days he could not work out how to use tools, even though he'd been a farmer all his life.'
>
> After sailing through tests for Alzheimer's, Charles was diagnosed with depression. His wife thought it was the funniest case of depression she'd ever seen. Eventually, after he was diagnosed with Pick's disease, he described not knowing whether he was wrong or right as being incredibly demeaning, since he'd always been self-confident.
>
> His wife was both relieved and devastated by the diagnosis. 'You go through a grieving process, but knowing what we are dealing with makes it easier to manage and live with. When he does something stupid, you can just shrug it off.'

People with an FTD may lose the ability to empathise, and may appear selfish and unfeeling. You may notice a loss of inhibitions, and behaviours such as swearing, shoplifting, sexual activity in public, or disregard for personal hygiene may increase. Inappropriate actions can include tactless comments, joking at the wrong moments, or being generally rude, even grabbing food off another person's plate.

They may develop routines or compulsive rituals such as handclapping, humming the same tune over and over, walking the same route day after day. They may overeat and/or change their food preferences (from sweet to savoury or vice versa).

Reduced language abilities may mean the person has difficulty finding the right words, loses grammar rules, lacks spontaneous conversation, uses many words with little content or out of context, and has weak, imprecise and uncoordinated speech. (See Chapter 13: Communication.)

Huntington's disease

Huntington's is progressive and hereditary. Previously included among the FTDs, it is now classified in its own right. It usually appears in adults aged between 35 and 50, and an early symptom is uncontrollable, rapid, jerky, body movements.

> Sean loved nothing better than a heated discussion. He had always waved his hands around as he talked, but then he and his family noticed a change. He would miss the table when putting a cup down, and his gestures were increasingly agitated. He stopped working. He continued driving very carefully (at 40 kph in the middle of the road); but he sold his boat because he realised he was unsafe in it.
>
> One day he collapsed after helping to push a broken-down car. In hospital he was linked up to various machines, made their signals jump all over the place and Huntington's disease was diagnosed. Sean was then in his mid-sixties. The family had no idea where this inherited disease had come from, although they pinpointed a grandfather reputed to be 'difficult'!
>
> The disease progressed quickly. Sean took no medicines, got up late, went to bed early, walked 'drunkenly' for a bit of exercise with good friends, had increasing difficulty in swallowing but didn't want any fuss. He was starting to say that he didn't want to go on, when he died quite unexpectedly less than a decade after his diagnosis.

Other early symptoms include: muscle spasms; progressive loss of memory, concentration, planning and organising skills; lack of insight into their condition; lack of concern for others' needs.

No specific treatment exists for Huntington's, but drugs may help control the muscle spasms. Those affected continue to recognise people and places, and need calmness and patience in those around them.

Early-onset dementia

Some people develop dementia – various kinds – in their forties, with rare cases coming even earlier. Few expect dementia in people younger than 60 or 65 and, given the stigma, hardly anybody would dare suggest it. If they see forgetfulness, inefficiencies at work, or poor running of a house and family, they are more likely to blame menopause, possible little strokes, or surreptitious drug or alcohol problems.

This is where society's discomfort with dementia really needs to change, as the sooner any available treatments are started, the better.

> One woman in her early forties struggled on working full-time and bringing up her teenage daughters while finding queer things happening in her life. She couldn't believe it when she was told she had early-onset dementia. She eventually had to stop working, but remained as positive as she could, and remarried a few years later a very supportive man.

Another challenge for people who develop dementia early in life is that dementia services, especially care facilities, are for the elderly and frail.

Where to from here

- Chapter 2: The Doctor and the Diagnosis
- Chapter 4: Dealing with the News
- Chapter 6: Becoming a Carer
- Chapter 15: Maintaining Health

Chapter 4

Dealing with the News

Reluctance to accept

If the person you are caring for is reluctant to accept their diagnosis, doesn't want to admit they have dementia and rejects outright the doctor's findings, try to find out why – but don't hammer them with questions. (See Chapter 13: Communication, and Chapter 12: Feelings). For instance, you could make an empathetic statement, such as: 'You really think there is nothing wrong'; 'You are frightened and hoping it will all go away'; or 'You're uneasy because there is dementia in your family background.'

If they continue to be adamant that there is nothing wrong with them, you will have to try another tack – but never argue. Strange as their behaviour may be, in their new state of mind it makes sense to them; or they may always have been accustomed to being in control; or perhaps this forcefulness is typical of their family.

Covering up

Your own first inclination may be to play down or even cover up the dementia when you are with others. This is a natural reaction.

> 'I think the first year you try to hide it, don't you?' said a wife. 'I'd answer for Frank if we were talking to somebody – you get over-protective, you stick up for your husband. When he couldn't get his words out I'd say them for him.
>
> 'My husband was taken into hospital for a prostate operation. When he was out of bed they couldn't find him. He'd wandered

off and that brought it out into the open. Once it was out it was a great relief.'

Denial is understandable if you or others want to avoid the stigma that is still associated with any illness affecting the mind. Maybe that is why one woman replaced the word 'dementia' with another that seemed more socially acceptable and less threatening:

> Beverley was told that her husband, George, had dementia. In a bit of a daze she remembered her old neighbour, Phyllis, whose husband had had Alzheimer's for years before he died; so she phoned Phyllis for advice and a friendly shoulder to lean on after the dementia diagnosis.
>
> After Beverley had poured out her anguish, Phyllis replied, 'But Dennis didn't have dementia, Bev. He had Alzheimer's.' Beverley felt very embarrassed.

Talking and planning together

One of the first things to do after the diagnosis is to talk over the bad news together – just you and the diagnosed person. If you are close to them, tell them how much you love them, have plenty of hugs, and remain as warmly affectionate as possible. As someone with dementia has said, 'We need support and comfort after we've been given what is one of the worst diagnoses anyone can get.' Be open about things and shed tears together. It's a tough prognosis. But sit down and start to plan. This gives you both positive goals to aim for. If you are not a close couple, or if you are a paid carer, you can still demonstrate warmth as you tell them that you want to form a coping team. In either event, set aside definite times to plan for the future.

The early stages of dementia are confusing and frightening, but you can both use the months ahead to make detailed and necessary plans for your financial security (see Chapter 5: Legal and Money Matters) and general plans for future care.

> Connie and Trevor were both stunned. They didn't know how they should react with each other over the diagnosis of Trevor's dementia. As they walked their dog to the park that afternoon

Connie held Trevor's arm, which she didn't usually do. She needed his support as much as she thought he needed hers.

Trevor said how lucky they were to live just across the road from a rest home, where he could go when he became bad enough. He phoned the Alzheimer's Society to join up.

Connie bought a book on dementia which Trevor (still able to read) leafed through, commenting that it did not seem to be him at the moment. Connie thought it was; he was exhibiting most of the first-stage symptoms, but she didn't tell him.

They spent a lot of time talking about the future and planned to go on living normally and to make the most of every day.

Together, discuss and decide how to tell your family. Also work out who you will tell among friends and workmates, and how you will tell them. Talk about the current job or other responsibilities of the person who has just been diagnosed and about your own commitments to employer, employees, and so on.

Talk to your family doctor together, and get in touch with Alzheimer's or other relevant societies. (See Chapter 2: The Doctor and the Diagnosis, 'Ideal ways to reach a diagnosis'; and Chapter 7: Dealing with Health Professionals, 'Your doctor'.)

If the newly diagnosed person refuses to be part of the 'planning team' and the steps discussed in this section, bring in a trusted family member or friend to discuss things with regularly.

Telling family members

Once you have both decided which family members should be told, decide how much to tell them about the situation and diagnosis. Work out how soon you can meet the people you have chosen – adults and children – to let them know your news.

On the agreed date, both of you meet with everyone together. Explain the diagnosis, the expected path and length of what is ahead, and all the details you know and have decided to share. Be ready and make time for lots of questions.

Some of your family may be aware of the mental deterioration, and some may be completely oblivious. To bring them all into the picture, recount a few 'funny' incidents to let them know what's been happening. These should let them understand that you may need their help, and make the meeting less threatening. Others have told their families:

> 'Your dad boiled up the tea bags in the kettle yesterday, and we thought it was time we told you that that was only one of the funny things that he's been doing. You may have to become our parents and look after us!'

> ✦

> 'Mum took two hours the other day to get to Jude's place – and you would know that Jude lives only five minutes away.'

> ✦

> 'Your sister bought the entire contents of the door-to-door-salesman's stock last month. I had a terrible job to persuade his company to destroy the contract and take them back!'

> ✦

> 'Your mother came home by taxi from her last shopping trip and told me her car had been stolen. She'd reported it to the police. The next day the car was found in the mall's parking lot.'

Answer the family's questions and discuss your aims. Try to accept any help that they offer. Research and experience have found that emotional or practical support works best when it comes from close friends or family members. Information and advice, on the other hand, are best coming from people considered to be experts. Ideally, your family should consult you about what you would find most helpful. (See Chapter 10: Wider Support and Self-care, 'How the wider family can help'.)

Whether the person with dementia acknowledges their condition or not, the family will soon be in the know, and you will have to cope with their reactions as well as your charge's condition. Sometimes their response will be entirely practical:

> One family had been shielded from their mother's dementia for years. They said later that, if they had known, they would have read up about the subject and given much more understanding and helpful support.

When their mother's long-suspected diagnosis was finally admitted they got together, pooled all their knowledge and experiences and then itemised their aims and plans: to keep their own sanity; to support their father (her main carer) as well as possible; and to keep their mother at home as long as possible.

Families can disagree

Some family members will be unable to agree on the prescribed dementia treatment for the person concerned, and often others will think it is their right or responsibility to offer, or even push, advice.

Sometimes, especially if the person with dementia lives alone and wishes to stay where they are, living arrangements will be a subject of debate. Some relatives will insist that the diagnosed person needs constant care now. Others will suggest that they are still the same as they were before the diagnosis and should be able to live the same way.

On the other hand, family members may think you, the carer, are exaggerating.

Heather, Godfrey's sister, had accused his wife of exaggerating Godfrey's loss of faculties and spreading untrue stories about him having dementia. When she came in from the country to stay, however, she seemed friendly enough and asked what she could do to help.

'Thanks. You could go to the supermarket and do some shopping for me,' Sheila replied. 'Take Godfrey along with you and start catching up on family news. He doesn't drive, you know, but he can push the trolley, can't you, darling?' she said to him.

'Too right,' he replied, and the brother and sister went together out the back door with the shopping list, some money and the car keys.

A minute later, as the car went slowly past the kitchen window, Sheila saw her husband in the driver's seat. She dashed out the front door and waved her arms to make him stop. 'I told you Godfrey didn't drive,' she called to Heather through the half-open car window.

'Of course he can drive,' Heather replied crossly. 'Look at him. He's driving, isn't he? Anyway, I'm here beside him so we can't come to any harm. Don't worry. Off you go, Godfrey,' she said, and they left Sheila standing as Godfrey drove off to the supermarket.

'You're happy to push the trolley for us?' Heather asked, as Godfrey drove in the car park gate.

'Yes, and I'll park as close as I can for you,' he replied. Before Heather could react, he drove up onto the footpath, along to the wide glass door entrance and through it, ending up parked amid shattered chaos right by the row of trolleys.

Heather's comments were not remembered for posterity. Sheila said, 'Well, I'm glad I didn't say he could get the ice cream for us. He might've tried to drive right round to that aisle!'

Some relatives may say, 'Mother is doing this on purpose,' when they think she has decided to be bloody-minded. They won't believe you when you say that this is just a sign of early dementia.

Alternatively, they may regard you as the cause of the problem, or even as the person who actually has the problem.

After Jonathan's wife, Sue, was diagnosed with Alzheimer's, he looked after her at home as carefully and patiently as he could, although at times he thought he would go bonkers. What really got up his nose was that one of his daughters accused him of mistreating Sue and causing her confused and sometimes odd behaviour.

He became so desperate he purposely arranged a week's business trip and asked that daughter to have her mother to stay while he was away. Only the day after he had left, the daughter phoned their family doctor, quite unable to cope with her mother, and pleaded for help.

She later apologised to her father and they were reconciled.

Telling friends and colleagues

You've told your family about the diagnosis, now for the others – friends, acquaintances and workmates.

You may want to be careful who you tell, keeping in mind that some people may not react positively. This may include talking about you behind your back and twisting the information; or simply failing to understand, and therefore getting the information wrong. Some people may say, 'Oh yes, I know so-and-so and they've got this too,' taking the focus away from your fateful message and carrying on about their own interests.

It is wise to be careful how you tell people too. You are both full of the shattering news you have been given, and may be tempted to detail all the symptoms you have experienced and how long you have kept quiet. Don't do this. Spare telling people all but the general details. Make a short list of what you will speak about, and cover these same points each time you bring someone into your confidence.

Once you tell your true friends, they will visit and support, or offer to spend time keeping your charge company while you go out – just 'dropping in' tactfully when you've asked them to (your charge won't want to be 'baby-sat'). As with the man in the following story, they may be flattered to be told.

> Noel and Bruce had been sporting rivals at different schools in their teens, and retained a mutual regard for each other in their late sixties. They still played tennis together.
>
> 'What's the matter with Bruce?' Noel had asked Alison one day, when Alison herself was wondering what was up with her husband.
>
> 'I don't know, Noel,' she replied. 'He's not his old self, is he?'
>
> Alison didn't tell Bruce about this conversation until after his Parkinson's and dementia diagnoses a few months later, when the two of them were discussing how to handle the bombshell with their friends. They decided that many other people might face similar nightmares as they got older, and that they should share the news around.
>
> Noel was one of the first they contacted. He was flattered to be told, although distressed by the news, and he provided sincere and regular support from then on. Bruce was relieved that he didn't have to put on any false fronts.

People who stay away

Dementia makes many people uneasy, at least initially. Fear that they may see a friend 'losing it' can lead some to put off visiting.

> All the members of Graeme's tennis group called in occasionally to see him after he started declining with dementia; all of them except one, who kept away because he said he couldn't bear to see his old friend deteriorating. Graeme was very hurt.

Friends and acquaintances may also stay away because they don't know what to talk about and how to behave. They may think you and your charge will be embarrassed if they come, or that they don't know you well enough for you to want to see them. Perhaps they decide they haven't the time. They may not even be clear to themselves (let alone you) about why they don't come.

> One man with dementia wrote that as soon as his diagnosis was announced some people became very uncomfortable around him. Gingerly, he sought people out who were avoiding him, told them he didn't bite, that he was still 'at home' in his head and that he needed their friendship and acceptance.

If people keep away, and you know them well enough, get in touch. Say how much of a gap they are leaving and ask if they could visit. They may be flattered by this, and glad you made the decision for them.

Telling employers

If the newly diagnosed person is still in a job, they may wish to remain employed for as long as possible. If they are the boss, they will probably have some control over the process – at least when it comes to disclosure.

> Helen said of her CEO husband, Donald, 'We certainly discussed the diagnosis, and he was particularly dignified and open about it all, telling his family, staff and friends himself, as he was keen to avoid chit-chat or incorrect information being circulated. People were generous in their sympathy and admired him for his honesty. Neither of us wanted it to be kept secret.'

However, an employee (and their carer) may want to think more carefully about how they deliver the news to the employer.

After Larry told his boss, he was shunted out of his position pretty quickly. 'Can't have accidents happening at work,' his boss said, although Larry was not on any production line where accidents could happen. He found himself very quickly in a sticky situation financially, and wished he had not been so open about his diagnosis. He thought about appealing, but didn't have the energy, nous or bank balance to risk it.

Larry may have needed a support person with him when he talked to his employer, or perhaps he didn't choose his words carefully enough. It is wise for the person with the dementia diagnosis to make three points:

1. They are still the person they were yesterday and can presumably still do the work they were doing then, until further notice.
2. They value their employment and wish/need to have an income while they make plans for the rather questionable future.
3. They will keep their employer informed about their progress.

In some cultures it may not be necessary to tell the employer. In China, for example, people may choose to retire from their forties onwards and still receive a good percentage of their wage or salary. You may decide on this path because your family will feel it is their duty to care for their elderly or sick dependant. Sending their parent to a rest home is not acceptable, as it will bring strong disapproval from their community. In many cultures families are committed to caring for old or sick relatives, and employers in these cultures are generally sympathetic to the employee's needs in these circumstances.

Where to from here

✦ Chapter 5: Legal and Money Matters
✦ Chapter 7: Dealing with Health Professionals
✦ Chapter 6: Becoming a Carer
✦ Chapter 8: Adapting the Home Environment
✦ Chapter 10: Wider Support and Self-care
✦ Chapter 11: Independence and Safety
✦ Chapter 12: Feelings
✦ Chapter 15: Maintaining Health

Chapter 5

Legal and Money Matters

The very first thing to do after a dementia diagnosis is to see a family lawyer and an accountant – even though this is probably the last thing you want to bother with at the time. Some people advise doing this even before you meet with extended family and friends to discuss your momentous news.

If you do not have a lawyer or accountant, look in a local business directory for names of those practising in your neighbourhood. Alternatively, check the listings of relevant professional organisations, such as law societies or chartered accountants' societies. Some countries have specialist groups of lawyers for the aged, with contact details for their members available on the internet, as well as in print. Ask acquaintances about the reputations of those whose names come up, and enquire from several sources, because word of mouth is usually the best gauge of approval.

If you can't afford a lawyer or accountant, voluntary organisations such as Citizens Advice Bureaux may have duty lawyers available for minor consultations, and a wide selection of material to help you. Free community groups such as Age Concern, Age UK or your national equivalent may be able to help. Community law offices, legal aid or the public trustee may also offer inexpensive or free advice. Some governments have agencies offering financial planning information on the internet and in brochures. Free non-governmental budgeting services are usually widespread as well. (See, for example, Useful Resources at the end of this book.)

Essentials to deal with immediately
Enduring powers of attorney

Many people think that simply being the spouse or next of kin gives them the right to act on behalf of a person who can no longer make informed decisions of their own. This is not the case. Another assumed 'right', the authority to sign on another person's bank account, is very limited and expires once a doctor certifies that the person with dementia is no longer mentally competent.

A power of attorney is a written document in which 'the nominator' authorises someone, 'the nominee', to make decisions on their behalf. Your charge may have had such a document drawn up and signed before their diagnosis, but it becomes null and void once they lose their mental ability.

So, while they are still legally competent (with mental capacity, or in their right mind), you and they need to arrange an enduring power of attorney (EPOA, known also as 'durable' or 'lasting' power of attorney). These exist until death, or until legally revoked by the nominator; but they only come into effect when activated by a doctor on a legal certificate verifying that the person is no longer competent.

In order to protect you and your charge, have your lawyer draft an EPOA. A diagnosis of dementia does not necessarily mean that your charge lacks mental capacity to sign these documents, but it is crucial that they sign while they still obviously have their wits about them.

> Elise had had a successful business career as well as marriage and four children. She and her husband supported each other staunchly through their ups and downs; and when she had a succession of TIAs (mini-strokes) in her seventies he was still supportive, as her short-term memory deteriorated and her behaviour became unpredictable.
>
> She refused any help, declaring – in her usual confident tones – that she was fine and on top of things, but she kept forgetting that she had had a drink and constantly returned to the gin bottle. Her husband quietly covered up her befuddled state.
>
> The family did not really notice her decline until their father himself had a severe stroke and they found out what he had been

coping with. They took it in turn to do what they could for a very uncooperative Elise, but financing both their parents' care began to drain their resources. Then they discovered they couldn't legally use their parents' funds, and were at their wits' end when their father died.

The family lawyer could do nothing either. 'An enduring power of attorney would have been the thing,' he said, 'but your father didn't have one and your mother has to be "of right mind" to be a signatory. We'll have to get a court order – but that will take a while.'

Two types – property and personal care

Many countries have two types of EPOA. One, a property EPOA, can cover property, commercial interests, donations, bank accounts, and so on. The other, a personal care and welfare EPOA, covers medical treatment, the type of accommodation and daily support, and so on.

For a property EPOA there may be several choices to consider:

- limiting it (for example to bank accounts and house) or leaving it broad – the latter means that you need not review the EPOA if assets change
- having it take effect immediately, or only when doctor signs the certificate
- arranging more than one nominee – this means you have checks and balances, and there is more likely to be someone on hand for a decision or signature.

The nominee for a property EPOA may or may not be the same individual as the personal care and welfare EPOA nominee.

A personal care and welfare EPOA is usually given to only one person (although it may name a substitute if the nominee is unable or unwilling to act). It may also be limited or broad in the aspects it covers, and usually takes effect only when the subject is certified as mentally incapable.

This kind of EPOA can affect the person with dementia significantly when a permanent change has to be made in their place of residence, such as entering full-time or hospital care, or undergoing a major medical procedure.

The choice of nominees for EPOA is therefore important. Despite the word 'attorney' it need not be an attorney or lawyer (if it is, they may invoice for acting on your charge's behalf). It must, however, be someone empathetic whom your charge can trust.

Most countries' laws protect the interests of people who are the subject of EPOAs; for instance, New Zealand has made legal changes to prevent undue pressure on vulnerable people who have signed these documents, and to ensure consultation. There are also restrictions, such as age and solvency, on who can be nominated as an attorney. Both the nominator and the nominees must sign and have their signatures witnessed.

Joint bank accounts

Arrange to have money in a joint bank account, so that you as carer can keep track of how your charge is using funds; or make arrangements with the bank for a second signatory on your charge's bank account for the same reason. This does not take the place of an EPOA, and like an EPOA it must be done while the person with dementia is still able to comprehend what powers they are granting.

Once your charge enters full-time care with a state subsidy it is better to have a separate bank account for them, since they may be means-tested to qualify for a benefit.

Wills

Check that both you and your charge have current and appropriate wills. For instance, if your spouse, family member or close friend is the person with dementia, you may want to change the beneficiaries named in your will. Setting up a trust may be one way to ensure that they benefit from your estate. If you want to leave a legacy for your charge, however, you may first need to know how this will affect any government benefits they draw.

When your charge updates or changes their will, it is important to involve the lawyer and to make sure they know about the dementia diagnosis. They may seek to check the person's mental capacity with a doctor, to avoid a later challenge to the wishes expressed in the will.

Assets and other financial factors

As dementia progresses, the person affected will increasingly be unable to manage their own finances, so confer with them while they are still in the early stages of the disease. If they are unable to engage or are uncooperative, consult with other advisers.

Identify all their assets: real estate, bank accounts, insurance policies, shares and so on. It is important to do this while they are still able to organise things and before any crucial records become lost or are inadvertently destroyed. List these assets, together with their current value and the names of any owners, account holders or beneficiaries. Provide the list to the lawyer – preferably before an EPOA is signed – and accountant, together with copies of any related official documents. Ask those professionals to examine carefully any property that your charge owns separately, with a view to putting it into joint ownership if necessary.

Survey your and your charge's present and future financial situation, state of insurances, and so on. Talk to a lawyer and/or accountant about the options you and your charge have for financing long-term care.

Consider arranging direct debits to pay bills for local government charges, power, telephone, water and other ongoing services. This will reduce confusion when posting cheques or using credit cards becomes difficult.

If possible, use suitable DVDs to inform your charge about new financial arrangements or investments and to give them a sense of still being involved. These can be viewed several times.

Protecting the carer

If your finances and those of your charge have always been combined, work with an accountant to restructure them so that you can draw on them after your charge dies. If their bank account covered daily living costs, their estate will be frozen when they die and paying regular bills can be almost impossible. Even after probate has been granted, household money in the not-yet-finalised deceased estate can be impossible to access.

Talk to your doctor, accountant or relevant government agency about any pensions or allowances for which you may be eligible as a carer.

Advance care directives

An advance care directive or 'living will' is an optional step, and is not legally binding. However, it can help the personal care and welfare attorney to make decisions or advise doctors of their charge's stated preferences. It states which health interventions (medications or procedures) the subject would or would not like, and sets out the circumstances. Before drawing up such a directive it is wise to get information from your doctor about interventions that are foreseeable and the consequences of having or not having them. As with an EPOA, the person with dementia must be mentally capable at the time of signing it.

Advance care planning

This may be the time to do advance care planning – a fairly new internationally recognised method of informing people about your wishes in the event of your becoming gravely ill or disabled. It allows you to give instructions for future health care, donation of organs and selecting your chosen physician.

Dealing with finances in the future

Having financial practicalities sorted out will help you to cope more easily with managing the dementia itself. Below is a checklist to ensure you have considered all the important questions. All these points can be discussed with your lawyer and/or accountant.

- Have you adjusted finances so that both you and your charge have independent incomes?
- Do you have sufficient capital available to invest and produce interest to pay expenses if you stop work to become a carer?
- What avenues are open for you to be paid as a carer?
- Do you need to call in life insurance policies or sell shares?
- Will you need to apply for government benefits?
- Have you factored possible sickness (yours or your charge's) and long-term care costs into your estimates?
- Will the surviving partner (you or your charge) be left with enough to live on?

If the person with dementia is your parent:
- ✦ Do they have assets that may help with costs and that you can access?
- ✦ How much financial help do you feel able to give your parent with dementia?
- ✦ How will your own plans be limited by giving them financial or other help?
- ✦ Will financial or other help from you diminish the grandchildren's inheritance?

The complexity of court orders

If you find yourself responsible for a person with dementia who is past making important decisions, who is unable to understand the courses you are proposing, cannot sign documents, and who has made no arrangements for enduring powers of attorney, the courts need to appoint someone to resolve these matters. This is expensive and can also be time-consuming and destructive to family harmony, since family members cannot always agree on who should be appointed. Avoid this situation if you possibly can.

Family issues

Financial help from family and friends can be a godsend at times; but it needs tact and honesty to enquire and to accept. You also need to be clear about any expectations the lender or donor may have as a result, and whether you can meet them.

There may be ructions involving children, stepchildren or other relations, over future powers of attorney, family trusts, the use of funds for outside caring, or the treatment of their loved one. Such altercations can be extremely distressing.

> Stephanie had been Greg's second wife for many years when he developed Alzheimer's. Although despondent, she felt secure and safe: she trusted and felt well advised by his lawyer, was a beneficiary in family trusts which took care separately of his offspring and her, and she knew that appropriate powers of attorney and other provisions were already in place for future needs. Then

suddenly Greg's son – an outsider with no visible means of support – chose to come back into their lives and spring into vicious action. He terrified her with physical threats, accused her of luring his father away and milking him financially, and he challenged the family trusts, in the process creating legal mayhem which began to deplete the family coffers at an alarming rate.

Not many family members will react in such a devastating way but some will wrangle incessantly. If they become really involved and obstructive, try to arrange a meeting with them and an independent counsellor or other facilitator. Experienced and empathetic doctors can sometimes help, if they have the time. It is important to find constructive help from somewhere outside the family. Without management and support, you can find that this sort of criticism shatters your health and confidence.

Where to from here

✦ Chapter 4: Dealing with the News
✦ Chapter 7: Dealing with Health Professionals
✦ Chapter 10: Wider Support and Self-care
✦ Chapter 11: Independence and Safety
✦ Chapter 25: Choosing Full-time Care
✦ Chapter 27: Final Days

Part Two

Making Adjustments

Chapter 6

Becoming a Carer

A different relationship

Until now, your life roles may have been as a son or daughter, school child, employee or employer, parent, husband or wife, partner or grandchild; now you have been catapulted into another – as a primary or secondary carer. Difficulties are normal where there are changes in roles.

The person you are caring for may feel resentment towards you, because you now make the decisions and they are not in control of their lives as they were before. You may be a previously submissive spouse taking care of your dominant spouse, or you may already be the dominant one of the two of you. You may be a 'child' becoming a 'parent', as in this story:

> When Doug began to develop dementia, Gloria, his wife, decided they should leave their long-loved home and move a long way to be near their son, Henry. She really pushed Doug into this and bought a suitable apartment. After they moved in, Doug complained non-stop. He threatened to move back 'home'.
>
> Gloria, and Henry's wife and family, all told him Doug was mad; but Henry listened to his father and identified with his feelings. Doug felt so relieved someone had at last understood that he grudgingly changed his mind.
>
> Henry, however, had not done this easily. He realised that he and his father had switched roles and he now had to parent his father.

Perhaps you, too, feel discomfort at your altered relationship – or perhaps you feel gleeful. There may be friction ahead; or your relationship may change for the better.

You and the person you are now looking after may have talked about these changing roles – or not. If you stumble over issues like this, try to resolve them openly, and find ways to start talking about them, with positive statements. (See Chapter 12: Feelings, 'Deal positively with your feelings'.)

> Henry gave his mother a break and deliberately took his father on one of his business trips. During this enforced togetherness, and with 'I' messages that a recent seminar had taught him to use, Henry told his father how uncomfortable he felt and why.
>
> To Henry's intense surprise, his father said he felt the same way. They had a long talk. Henry clarified anything his father said that he didn't understand, and discovered that his father was still sharp in many areas, despite the dementia. They began to rebuild their relationship.

Your reasons for becoming a carer

If you are becoming a major carer for someone with dementia, it is a good idea to analyse why. Firstly, the person may be your long-loved partner, parent or sibling for whom you are undertaking the new task willingly – even if it involves changing roles with them (for instance, they could previously have been the dominant one in your team).

Secondly, the person could be someone with whom you don't get on well, and you are going to care for them from a great sense of duty, or because culturally it is expected of you. In this case you may wish to be relieved of the role as soon as possible, but good on you for taking it on in the meantime.

Thirdly, the carer role may give you a place to live, and/or payment for work. You may either find a new career opening in front of you, or discover it is not for you. Either way you will learn a great deal and become much wiser.

No matter what your reasons are for becoming a carer, it is wise to seek out some specific knowledge or training to help you.

Review how you operate

It is also important to examine your coping skills honestly, for instance by looking through the following 10 statements and choosing between the options in bold that suit your style:

1. As a carer, I am **strong/anxious**.
2. I will, as much as possible, **let my charge look after themselves/ protect my charge**.
3. I **will/won't** discuss dementia matters with my charge.
4. In communicating with the doctor I will **talk openly/censor my reports to maintain my charge's dignity**.
5. I will **join appropriate organisations/cope by myself (organisations are for others)**.
6. On my own or when socialising, I eat and drink **moderately/to excess**.
7. It is important to **lower my expectations of my charge and myself/ keep up high standards**.
8. I want to **know the course of this disease/take it as it comes**.
9. I will manage **as a team with my charge/my charge to prevent them becoming a nuisance to me or others**.
10. I can see myself **caring for my charge in a practical way with love/ already veering towards dislike for my charge**.

If you have ticked the second option in several statements above, or if you already feel agitated or unsure, you may find being a carer difficult or overwhelming. Your charge may be better off with another family member or a paid full-time carer, or in full-time care, than with you being grumpy or overwrought.

Hard work and getting help

Caring for someone with dementia is hard work, especially in the later stages. These develop gradually, however, and with help, you can manage reasonably satisfactorily until you need to consider full-time care.

From the moment of diagnosis, look into every avenue for advice and help. These may come from your family, family doctor, specialist, organisation's support workers, hospital staff and others (see Chapter 7: Dealing with Health Professionals, 'Other help from the health industry').

Be aware, too, that you may be eligible for quite a lot of free support. If your charge is a beneficiary in the hospital system, you could have help for example with showering and dressing, housework, gardening and the installation of equipment for assisting the disabled.

Keep on learning about the condition you are dealing with so that you can be ready for the next symptoms that may appear. Consult all possible authorities; but, if you use the internet for information, be aware that it may contain inaccuracies or unwise advice.

As your charge's personality and needs change, take care that you don't reject help from professional support people because you think it is inappropriate, not good enough, coming at the wrong time, offered in a careless fashion or leaving you with little control. If you do have problems with professional support people, the reasons may vary: they may not have completed training; paid caregivers may be on low wages; personalities may clash; or the help may not be offered in a way that makes it easy for you to accept. Such a situation is not easy, but it is not insoluble.

Speak with your doctor, the support person's supervisor, your health care provider, a counsellor, or even a community advisory organisation such as a Citizens Advice Bureau. You may be assigned another professional support person, or perhaps the difficulties you are experiencing can be dealt with through problem-solving skills. (See Chapter 12: Feelings, 'Problem-solving'.)

Try not to feel guilty when at times you hate being a major carer or get totally fed up with the situation. Ring up your friends and unburden yourself to them occasionally (not too often!). It is not being disloyal to the person you are looking after. Also, many such confidants may eventually have someone close to them with dementia, and these stories will one day help them cope.

Know your limits, and refer often to the Carer's Code (see Chapter 10: Wider Support and Self-care).

Regularity, routine and organisation

Doing the same thing at the same time every day – for example breakfast, shower, dressing, sitting in same chair, sandwiches for lunch – makes life run more smoothly as the dementia becomes more pronounced. Always keep everything in the same place: sunglasses, mobility taxi card, tea bags, instant coffee and biscuits. This enables your charge to help themselves more easily.

At some point they will be unable to deal with more than one action at a time. They may say, for example, 'I can't talk and walk upstairs at the same time' or 'I can't walk and carry a cup' – or you yourself may notice this. Allow enough time for them to do things at their own pace, and try to see they don't get overloaded. It is wise to ration your own energy, too, and aim to have no more than one extra activity a day for your charge.

If you avoid mentioning future engagements until just beforehand, they can't get agitated about what time they have to be ready to leave. Do, however, continue the routines they have become used to.

> Stacey went on regularly taking Ernest to films and concerts and outings to friends' homes. She took him to watch his old mates play their regular tennis and bowls games, or to have lunch at his golf club, or to a local restaurant for dinner.
>
> Her son said, 'Why, Mum? It's hard, hard work for you, getting Dad and his walker into the car and out again, and he looks such a wreck. He drops food everywhere. Why don't you just keep him at home?'
>
> Stacey shook her head. 'Just imagine yourself in Dad's place. Life's awfully dull sitting at home all the time. It's been his normal life, to go out in this way, so why shouldn't he continue? Sure, it can be a bit embarrassing, and he does look untidy and terribly disabled as he gets round the place, but he wants to do these things. Why shouldn't he? And when his friends ask him to join them, why shouldn't he accept?'

Reminding and recording

As your life becomes more complicated as a carer, and your charge's memory becomes increasingly unreliable, reminder notes and records will become more important.

Events calendar tips

- If your charge wants to do small tasks and can still read, write down the steps on a large card, in large, clear, dark printing.
- List 'things to be done' or appointments for the next few days on a prominently hung calendar.
- If your charge is computer-literate, use an email system as a memory aid for appointments or tasks to be followed up. Check emails every morning.
- Nine out of 10 times it's okay to remind your charge about something.

Life book

Start a life book for your charge – for the future, and for when they are with other carers who don't know them well. They will probably be chuffed to help you compile it.

This scrapbook can be in any form you wish, but use quality paper, because it may be well thumbed through. Fill it over months and years, with help also from the wider family, with photos, memorabilia and details of life going back to their early days. Build it up with material on the following themes:

- childhood/adolescence/young adult/middle age/later age
- important people in their life, memorable events and special places
- hobbies, sports and interests, favourite foods, likes and dislikes, and so on.

Medical folder

Another essential is a folder containing your charge's medical records. Buy a spring-clip folder with 20 to 40 clear-plastic file envelope pages. Begin by inserting details of their:

- full name and address
- date and place of birth
- blood group
- health system ID.

Add any other information that hospitals need when a patient is admitted.

This should include details of all their known medical conditions and a list of all medicines, dates started, dosage information and what the medicines are for – whether prescribed medications or over-the-counter products, such as:

- skin lotions
- natural remedies
- dietary supplements
- painkillers
- laxatives
- cold medications.

The medical folder should have copies of all your charge's other medical records, such as blood and urine tests, and X-rays. Include, too, any hospital records handed out after discharge from previous admissions.

Emergencies do occur in the lives of people with dementia, and you will be grateful for the instant availability of this background information at various times. It's amazing how quickly the folder will fill up. Keep it in a handy place and show relevant contents to doctors, ambulance people, and so on, or have it to take to hospital if necessary.

Personal journal

One of the most beneficial weekly or daily perks you can give yourself is to keep a personal journal. Even if writing doesn't come easily to you, it can be a therapeutic exercise. Your journal can be a safety valve and your bible of information for future reference. It can also give you material for the consideration of doctors and other carers. Here are some ideas to get you started:

- buy a hardback notebook especially for the purpose
- record noteworthy events that occur – at any hour, in any day or week – and how they affect you
- write about your fears, frustrations and feelings
- date your entries.

Write in front of the person you are looking after; and talk about what you are writing – with sensitivity. They may be interested, and it may help them. If it upsets them, well, don't do it in front of them.

Learn acceptance

People with dementia can't learn through experience, so don't try to instil new information and expect them to act on it later. Don't blame your charge for not being able to do things they used to do, either. You would not blame someone who had a broken arm if they could not do certain things.

> Carey couldn't bear it when his bright academic wife Ruth became hesitant and made foolish statements after she was diagnosed with Alzheimer's. He constantly pointed out her mistakes, and she began withdrawing from him. Their family doctor saw what was developing and had a serious discussion with Carey, explaining what was going on in Ruth's brain. 'From now on Ruth is always right, no matter what she does,' Carey decided, and their relationship became much better.

As a general rule, accept almost any behaviour. If your 'friend' insists that they want to go home, and doesn't believe you when you tell them that they are there already, you could put them in the car and take them for a 10-minute drive, then tell them, 'Here we are. We're home!' as you reach your door again.

This works sometimes. But it won't work if they were thinking of their childhood home. You can't take them there. Instead, sit with them and let them talk about that childhood home. Listen, listen, listen. Perhaps get out that old, old photo album. Make a note of their nostalgic longing in your journal. If it happens often, note down what you did that coped with it successfully or unsuccessfully. Reference to these notes may help you next time.

Avoid contradiction

You can no longer say 'You should…' to a person with dementia. Their disease is in charge. They are not purposefully being hurtful or annoying. Try not to take anything personally. Instead, read widely to increase your understanding of your charge's occasionally strange behaviour. As the following story shows, it makes sense to them:

> Sitting in a doctor's crowded waiting room, a mother who had Alzheimer's asked 'Has our flight been called yet?' She'd been an

avid traveller and made sense of the crowd by assuming they were in a departure lounge. Her daughter didn't try to put her right. She said, quite off the cuff, that their luggage had been checked in, and the older woman visibly relaxed.

From this, and with professional help, Penny Garner (the daughter) developed a strategy for dealing with dementia, SPECAL, which stands for Specialised Early Care for Alzheimer's. Core ideas in this approach are:

+ don't ask questions
+ don't contradict
+ learn to love repetition (in questions asked and routines followed).

Another SPECAL aim is to adopt a primary theme from the past life of the person with dementia: an area in which they have been interested or had skills, and which will help them make sense of the present in a pleasurable way.

> For one woman with dementia the primary theme came from a well-worn, much-loved pair of ballet shoes. Her family was able to persuade her to rest by saying her feet must be sore from dancing, and could encourage her to get dressed by suggesting she was preparing for a performance. The woman became happier, more relaxed and less anxious. Later, when she could no longer live at home, her routines were successfully adopted by staff at her nursing home.

✦

> For a man with brain damage the primary theme was athletics. Stephen had been a national representative athlete 60 years before he suffered a brain injury which left him with gentle dementia and stiff limbs. Lillian overcame this by telling him, 'Time to relax like in athletics, Stephen,' as she herself demonstrated what she wanted. It made dressing him much easier.

Some people believe the rigid application of SPECAL can be deceptive and disempowering for the person with dementia. However, by using these ideas in moderation, you can make life easier for your charge. It is very stressful to have one's sense of reality constantly challenged by questioning or contradiction. People with dementia have said:

If we see or smell something that isn't there, don't feel you have to explain that we are imagining it. Listen comfortably. For us it is real.

♦

Don't try to help us remember something that just happened. If it never registered, we are never going to be able to recall it!

♦

Talk to us without questions. We get uneasy, uncomfortable and upset when we can't answer.

Times to ask, discuss and resolve

At times it can be helpful to ask questions of your charge. The following are sufficiently broad to relieve stress in someone with dementia rather than exacerbate it.

- ♦ 'If I could change one thing to make things better for you today, what would that be?'
- ♦ 'Now you're at this stage – what things do you need to do?'
- ♦ 'Right, now how can I help you the most?'

Making a contract

Soon after diagnosis, you and your charge will probably have talked about family or business matters and made realistic plans about the future, but things change.

If new problems arise, discuss them with the person you are looking after, write out any agreed solutions, and both sign. This can be useful even for what an outsider might view as minor domestic matters:

Susanne, aged 80, had helpers coming in each morning to shower and dress her husband Gilbert, who had dementia. They were very popular with her, but not with him. He became stroppy when they could not give a definite time of arrival.

'I can't wait for them,' he'd grumble. 'I like to get dressed first thing in the morning and, anyway, I don't like complete strangers coming in and washing me.' He would go secretly into the bathroom and make an awful mess trying – usually unsuccessfully – to shower and dress himself.

Susanne finally got very cross with him. 'I can't be clearing up after you any more, Gillie,' she burst out, 'and I usually end up having to dress you, which is very difficult now. I need help to look after you, and you're not helping me. It's unfair. I don't know how long I can go on. I am 80, you know. I'm jolly well going to get you to sign an undertaking. In return for me looking after you at home, you'll jolly well stay in your dressing gown every morning until they arrive, and that's that!'

It was so unlike Susanne to lose her temper that Gilbert meekly put his almost indecipherable signature alongside hers at the bottom of the contract she scribbled. It did help. Sometimes he forgot, and she had only to wave the paper at him and he would grumblingly do as she asked.

Dealing with fear

Fear can be a major factor in living with dementia, as people with the condition have commented themselves:

> I'm terrified. I'm absolutely terrified. My great terror is that the day will come when I forget everything. I may even forget when it's time to get up and when it's time to go to bed. I'm terrified of doing wrong.

Night-time and darkness in particular can produce hallucinations, terror and much agitation:

> Perhaps the first change I noticed was fear – at night in the total blackness, these fears I had never really known before come.

What does not seem real to you will seem very real to your charge, and vice versa, so acceptance rather than dismissal is important:

> If we say we are frightened, accept our fears – don't tell us not to be silly, that you are there to look after us. Our fears are very real and can dominate us.

If your charge seems afraid, you can start to address this by finding out the reason and any basis for their fear. Examining their environment is a good first step.

They may now be frightened or upset by a large person striding into the room, or by a person from another culture – especially someone in their native dress. Sounds may also startle and mystify. A person with dementia can find it hard to tell where a sound is coming from, and may look in all the wrong directions. The 'people' arguing in the next room may be television actors.

Companionship and time for yourself

To minimise both isolation and a sense of forced togetherness, seek a balance between companionship and 'time out' – for yourself and your charge. One common experience for carers is that their charge keeps following them around. If this happens to you, try to put up with it. They could be feeling insecure, and you are their anchor. You need your space, however, so admit this to yourself, and allow for it. Arrange to go out regularly so that your absence is part of daily routine.

People with dementia also commonly think they don't need to be 'baby-sat' or looked after – even if they do. A very fearful person may clearly need company in the evening but insist on staying in their own home, where officially they live alone.

For your own sake and theirs, when you want time out for yourself or if you feel you may explode, arrange for someone they know to drop by. Try to make their arrival seem like a coincidence, as though they have 'simply turned up'. 'Great,' you might say. 'I was just going out for a while. You two can have a catch-up while I'm out.' Church or volunteer groups may assist if friends are in short supply, you can't afford a paid helper, and the person you are caring for isn't yet classified as needing it.

Where to from here

✦ Chapter 8: Adapting the Home Environment
✦ Chapter 10: Wider Support and Self-care
✦ Chapter 11: Independence and Safety
✦ Chapter 12: Feelings, especially 'Problem-solving'
✦ Chapter 13: Communication
✦ Chapter 14: Intimacy, Love and Sex
✦ Chapter 25: Choosing Full-time Care, especially 'A carer's ongoing involvement'
✦ Chapter 26: Moving into Full-time Care, especially 'Your role changes'

Chapter 7

Dealing with Health Professionals

In the years ahead you and the person you are looking after will want accessible and empathetic doctors – people in whom you have confidence, and with whom you feel comfortable. For your part you need to be willing to ask questions of people in the health system, and to stand up for yourself and your charge.

> I should have been more assertive. Most of us tend to treat doctors, nurses and hospitals with great respect and back down in the face of possible disagreement. One piece of advice I would give to any carer is 'Be assertive.'

Your doctor may be supportive and helpful, but their time is usually too full to be able to give you a constant listening ear. This is why you need a good family member or friend as your main support.

Your doctor

Ideally your family doctor will have a good knowledge of both geriatric care and the various forms of dementia. In practice, however, you may end up knowing a great deal more than they do, and have to educate them about the symptoms you are dealing with and the day-to-day management you are involved in.

They will lead the management of your charge's condition – unless you, or the person you are looking after, have definite ideas about how to tackle it. Certainly your doctor will be responsible for general medical care. They need to be alert for other medical conditions and to provide

or oversee such standard services as:
- annual flu injections
- regular blood pressure checks
- blood tests
- prescriptions for medications.

Take responsibility yourself for making appointments for the checks above, however. Note too that although your doctor can prescribe all medications, including those originating with specialists, you are responsible for requesting repeat prescriptions when they are running low.

Abilities and knowledge

Part of being a good family doctor is the ability to give practical as well as medical advice. Your doctor should be aware of, understand and anticipate the stresses ahead for you as carer, and they need to be skilled in communicating with a person who has dementia. Your doctor should also have good knowledge of the support services that are available, and be able to coordinate these services when needed.

Of course doctors are not perfect. Some are competent, balanced and supportive, while others may seem fearful or aggressive – or they may simply be tired.

The doctor–patient relationship is an important one, and if you find your doctor is unsympathetic or you feel they do not properly understand your circumstances or do not have enough experience with dementia, you can change doctors. You do not have to stay with a doctor you are uncomfortable with.

> Because of fears about her mother's deteriorating mental condition, Julia had contacted Social Welfare. They told her that, to get services for an elderly person, it was best to work through a doctor. But Julia found her mother's doctor incredibly remote. As Julia told this woman doctor how distressing she was finding the state of affairs, and began to weep during the appointment, the doctor remained aloof. She simply remarked that she supposed it must be upsetting ... but offered nothing in the way of real comfort or advice.

Julia thought she couldn't change to another doctor, that she had to use her mother's – quite a natural assumption. But this is not the case: you can choose to see a different doctor, even if this brings a long-standing doctor-patient relationship to a close. You also have the right to seek a second informed opinion. Always do this if you feel unsure about your doctor's decision.

Making a choice

Think about your usual approach to your doctor. If you feel able to talk openly about your own health and that of the person you are looking after, you probably have a good relationship. If you are uncomfortable with the doctor's manner or sense they may not have dealt enough with dementia to provide all the necessary care:

- ask them whether they would rather you went to another practitioner with more experience of dementia
- use friends and word of mouth (or a dementia-related organisation) to help you choose someone else who can give you the service you want, or
- decide you are comfortable with them and they can learn with you and be part of your team.

Sharon found her usual doctor not at all aware, knowledgeable or helpful after Warwick was diagnosed with dementia. 'Find another doctor you trust,' she advised other carers, 'and go with your patient when they have an appointment. You have to have help available when and where you need it. You may or may not get it from friends and family. Make sure you've got an empathetic and helpful doctor!'

How you can help your doctor

Keep in regular touch with your doctor and medical team. The information you provide will help them assist both of you. Confer with your charge before going in to any doctor's appointment with them: two pairs of ears and two memories are better than one.

Use your journal to keep notes on your charge's condition and your own. Do this between appointments, and definitely when you feel strain beginning to take its toll. Be 100 per cent honest in every area of these notes, and include the little, apparently unnecessary details and any significant – even apparently insignificant – changes. Take your journal, or notes from it, to your appointments to help your doctor or specialist understand, diagnose and prescribe more precisely for both of you. Your journal will prove invaluable in these circumstances.

Don't be too proud to admit anything you may have forgotten or done wrong. You will feel better for unburdening yourself, and the doctor will be clearer about the situation.

Sometimes other family members (such as adult offspring) can struggle to find a way to enter the formal support network. This can be an issue if they are concerned about the charge and/or the caregiver.

When there is a gap in the doctor's knowledge about your charge's specific dementia, encourage them to seek the information on the spot from an authority. Show your willingness to learn: ask your doctor about books on your charge's condition.

Appointments

You will usually need double-length doctor's appointments, because your charge thinks and talks slowly and may have complex health issues. Remember, though, that these are appointments for the person you are looking after. Let them be the focus of the appointment and do their own talking – however slowly. Try not to take over, interrupt or talk for them. Just be available if they need you.

Go to any medical appointment with:
- their medical folder
- notes from your journal
- a list of worries, queries and comments.

Leave spaces by each item to write any answers. If you find some of your questions embarrassing, write them out for the doctor. Include useful information you have noted since last time. Make sure you include any symptoms or conditions you have noticed, regardless of their connection with dementia.

Going to the doctor alone

Go alone if you need to talk privately with the doctor about dementia issues. If necessary, use some personal health problem as an excuse to go on your own. Perhaps take along a trusted acquaintance who can remember things you may forget. Ask for second or third opinions elsewhere, if your doctor seems to be hedging.

Before a first visit on your own, ask that your charge's notes be available for reference, so the doctor is aware of your needs.

If the doctor declines to give you information because of privacy laws, and won't be persuaded by your power of attorney, ask your charge to sign a short note authorising them to speak openly with you. If they won't or can't do this, ask your mental health authority for a note to this effect. Be especially emphatic if you think more may be going on inside the demented brain than is apparent to the doctor. Admit you are not sure. Be open with the doctor about your concerns and don't underplay them. Describe as many symptoms as you can. They are no one's fault.

If you feel your doctor does not take you seriously, be assertive and press for a frank discussion. You, if you are the principal carer, need to know. It is not disloyal to want an explanation of any unusual behaviour.

Seeing a specialist

In the process of diagnosis or later, your doctor may refer your charge to a specialist such as a neurologist or geriatrician. Most specialists tend to prefer to see patients earlier in their illness rather than later, so, if your doctor doesn't raise the possibility, ask for a referral. It is comforting to consult someone with specialised knowledge, and important to have a full assessment. This makes for maximum accuracy in diagnosis, and can rule out whether the symptoms are caused by something that is reversible.

You probably know your charge better than anyone, so it may be a good idea to send the specialist a concise letter before your first appointment, setting out your observations, thoughts and questions. This may add valuable material to your doctor's referral letter, and better prepare the specialist. If you do write a preliminary letter, take a duplicate to your appointment and take notes of the specialist's replies. The specialist should also be happy to speak with you on the phone before or after an appointment, but ask permission from your person with dementia first.

Some people are intimidated by specialists and even by family doctors. If you are, try a new approach and think of them as team members. These medical people are human beings too. They want to help you.

Should you go private or public?

A private specialist can be expensive, but under a public hospital system, your charge may immediately be referred to a specialist at no cost. If you arrange an initial private appointment with the specialist of your choice, they may agree to put your charge on their public hospital list in the future, but be prepared for a long wait.

Referral to a specialist in the hospital system may not give you an appointment with the one you had hoped for or requested, but note that public hospitals usually employ the best practitioners, so go to them with confidence. If the 'chemistry' is not right with the person you are assigned to, you can explain and request a change after the initial appointment.

Memory clinics, mental health

Referral to a private memory clinic may also be acceptable: in the early stages of dementia this will often result in more in-depth testing, a more thorough assessment and an earlier diagnosis. Many people with dementia will be involved with mental services for older people.

Questions to ask

Ask at reception about the specialist's policies on fees and insurance (if seeing them privately) and on missed appointments. It pays to ask your specialist what experience they have with dementia. Other useful questions, for which you will of course find your own polite words, include:

- ✦ How familiar are you with my charge's dementia?
- ✦ How do you view your role in treating this patient? Ongoing or…?
- ✦ Do you mostly listen or talk? (You will soon find out!)
- ✦ Will you be talking to our usual doctor about coordinating care?
- ✦ How often should we see you?

Some of these may seem impertinent, but, tactfully handled, should elicit useful information and respect from the person on the other side of the desk.

Other help from the health industry

An occupational therapist will visit and assess daily living activities in your home and arrange for helpful equipment (see Chapter 8: Adapting the Home Environment for some suggestions). Physiotherapists provide mobility assessment, massage, simple exercises and aids which can be useful as your charge becomes frailer.

Ask your family doctor or the hospital for referrals to these and other experts, and arrange regular contact with them. Sometimes you may need to be assertive, or ask more than one person.

> The hospital made sure that Kristen had someone visiting each week day to wash and dress her husband, Clarry, after he had a stroke and developed vascular dementia; but 11 years later she was still plugging on with no more home help than that. She had no family around her. She had never had a break or a holiday. Her inefficient and vague doctor said he didn't know of any help available in the community, after she enquired. Years later she learned that she could have asked the hospital for a needs assessor and coordinator for more help with Clarry's case.

Needs assessors

The health system should have competent people in its ranks whose job it is to look after the needs of people with dementia. Such a person assigned to you will become a constant and necessary coordinator for your affairs. They can suggest and arrange regular assessments of your charge by doctors, specialists and themselves, and detect times when you need a break. Make sure you form a strong communication bond with them. It is important to have them working on your behalf before you reach the end of your tether, or before the condition of the person you are looking after becomes precarious.

As part of the hospital system, they can be very busy. This means you may have to wait a long time for an appointment, and longer before they can provide or install the help and equipment you need. Ask whether you may have copies of their ongoing notes and/or care plans to add to your medical folder. They and their team should survey the progress of the dementia every year or two. They will increase your 'ration' of hours of free assistance when these are obviously needed.

Day and respite care

The help you are allocated should cover day care. Look around for a recommended day-care facility where your charge can spend these allocated hours on one or more days a week. Some places pick up and return their charges; others need them to be 'delivered'. Usually the staff will look after people in a mixed-gender group of manageable size. Lunch, entertainment and afternoon tea are often provided.

Much later you will become eligible for 'respite care'. This is residential care for your charge, enabling you to have time out. Your health-care team's specialist in providing this care tells you how to prepare – what clothes, medications and other items to send – and together you select the most suitable-sounding facility of those available. Your choices are often limited to the beds made available for this purpose in the hospital system. Your local dementia organisation will answer most of your queries.

When full-time, permanent care has to be addressed, you will want to enquire about assessment by the Older People's Health Team (part of the hospital service).

Reducing the charges

After notching up a number of visits to doctors and other health professionals, in some countries you may be entitled to a card that reduces charges for some future services and prescriptions. Your doctor probably needs to sign the application form for this. A support organisation you may have joined for people with dementia may suggest other ways to receive help.

Your pharmacist

As you select your doctor, you also need to select your pharmacist carefully, because you may see them frequently.

The acetylcholinesterase inhibitors (AChEIs) that are prescribed for some people with Alzheimer's or Lewy body dementia are expensive if they are not government-subsidised. Pharmacists, however, go out of their way to develop good relationships with their customers; therefore, if you are going to be a very regular customer, shop around to negotiate the best price.

> Most of the men whose wives were in our support group were on several medications, and everyone moaned about the gigantic cost of one special prescription not funded through any state or government agency. We finally compared the prices we were paying and discovered wide discrepancies. One astute member had found a soft-hearted pharmacist who sold her the prescribed drug at a-still-high-but-almost-cost price. We all left that lunch meeting resolved to bargain with our own pharmacists.

As well as dispensing medications and giving advice about them, your pharmacist can dispose of unwanted medicines safely. They can also be useful:

- showing you how to use specialised devices like inhalers, nebulisers and blood glucose meters
- obtaining mobility aids not provided by your occupational therapist
- helping you stock your first aid kit.

They can also differentiate between major and minor problems, and help you to treat the latter, for instance dressing wounds.

Where to from here

- Chapter 2: The Doctor and the Diagnosis
- Chapter 6: Becoming a Carer, especially 'Medical folder' and 'Personal journal'
- Chapter 8: Adapting the Home Environment
- Chapter 10: Wider Support and Self-care
- Chapter 15: Maintaining Health

Chapter 8

Adapting the Home Environment

As the months go by, the need to reorganise your home may become obvious. Consider these initial suggestions and ask your occupational therapist or your dementia organisation about others.

Outside

Keep decks, patios, driveways and paths in good repair and free of moss. Install handrails on potentially slippery or icy paths outside the house, and have a ready supply of sand or salt to sprinkle on these paths.

Have ramps built over steps to make them easier for people with mobility problems or wheelchairs. You may be able to obtain community funding for these through your needs assessor or other support worker.

Inside
Things that can break

Try to make sure that direct routes through the house do not involve windows, or anything precious you wouldn't want broken. Sometimes people run uncontrollably and fall, especially those with Parkinson's disease dementia or Lewy body dementia.

> Once Alan broke from his shaky, short-step LBD walk into a run he couldn't stop himself. One night he began to run in the hall and continued along the hall, through the bedroom door and on until he fell, crashing down between a chair in the far corner of the room and the windows beside it.

His elbow shattered the window, but luckily the curtains were drawn and he wasn't cut. He was mightily shocked, however, realising that he could have fallen through the glass onto the stone terrace one floor below. He made sure that the chair was placed further over, to stop him if it happened again.

Think about removing mirrors on walls. These could certainly break, but additionally a person with dementia may see themselves in the mirror and be disturbed by the 'stranger' in the house.

Other safety precautions

Put a gate at the top of stairways both inside and outside the house. In stairways, make sure that banisters are strong and that steps have non-skid treads. Install handrails on both sides of any stairs, even if there are only one or two steps.

Keep rooms light and bright. This makes everyone more cheerful as well as lighting the way.

Also for safety, have smoke alarms installed. Fire station staff may fit them for older people.

Labels and locations

Label often-used objects around the house, for example 'Tea', 'Coffee', 'Fridge'; also label locations such as drawers or cupboards with 'Socks', 'Underwear' and so on, as appropriate. You'll be surprised how often this helps. Put 'Bathroom', 'Bedroom', 'Kitchen' and other notices on doors, so that the person with dementia can find them if they become lost.

Keep more than one

Have duplicate house and car keys cut. You never know who might forget where they are or put them somewhere unexpected.

Keep several boxes of tissues around the house. You can grab them instantly in the event of a minor spill or accident.

It would be wise to put a duplicate copy of your charge's list of medications in your wallet or purse, just in case. (See Chapter 6: Becoming a Carer, 'Medical folder'.)

Useful phone numbers, notes, instructions

Make a list of frequently used phone numbers in large print on durable white card. You can program some models of phone with single-digit codes so your charge need only punch in one number. Place the cards prominently by the most-used phones, together with contact details for ambulance, doctor and other services you may need in emergencies.

When you go out – something you will need to do regularly – leave a prominent note saying where you are going, who you are with, and when you will be home.

Living areas
Furniture

Fix or replace wobbly furniture. Lend your fragile, light pieces of furniture to your friends or family and acquire sturdier stuff.

> Selwyn had difficulty judging distances (a symptom of Parkinson's disease-related dementia). He tried to sit down on the arm of his chair one night, but slipped off onto the glass-topped table beside it. Of course the glass shattered and he suffered multiple but, luckily, mainly minor cuts to his hands. The first aid kit was very useful!

Your occupational therapist can arrange for your charge's favourite armchair to be placed on an adjustable platform so they can get into and out of the chair more easily. Have a phone within easy reach of this chair, with phone numbers handy.

At floor level

Change the finish on highly polished, slippery floors, or carpet them instead. Provide clear pathways through the house. Remove anything that could trip somebody up, such as small floor mats and rumpled carpets.

> An old girlfriend from Bruce's teenage years came with her husband to visit Bruce. As he came out eagerly to greet them, his toe caught on a small mat in the front hall and he tumbled to the floor. He wasn't hurt. As she helped him up, his wife, Alison, said cheerfully, 'Well, that's the second time Bruce has fallen for you, Jean!'

Shoes, newspapers, low tables and stools that could get in the way should be removed too, but in passageways chairs can make useful rest stations.

Cables and heating

Keep lamp cords and television and computer leads well out of the way. A product from your electrician or hardware store can turn a jumble of leads into one fat coil.

Cover thermostats for central heating, as your charge may fiddle with them. Make sure heaters (gas or electric) have strong safety guards, and hook your fire screen to the hearth surround, or fix a chest-high fireguard. It can be a useful leaning post for a person with dementia who is tired of sitting.

> Owen fell twice on to the empty hearth and was unable to hoist himself up. Pauline had to phone the St John's Ambulance for help. She wondered whether he would have moved himself if there had been a fire in the grate!

The kitchen
The stove-top and oven

Make sure pot handles are always turned towards the centre of the stove. Turn electricity off at the wall after using the stove or oven. Consider having a cover made for the stove, too, if it has a flat glass top which retains heat for a while after use. Remove knobs from element controls at night; most will just pull off.

Consider obtaining a gas detector, in case your charge turns on the gas without lighting the flame. Alternatively, think about having only electric appliances.

Water temperature

To prevent scalding, lower the thermostat on your hot-water tank to 60 degrees Celsius. This is for the water in the cylinder itself. The temperature for water that comes out of the tap is determined by a tempering valve, which should be set at 55 degrees Celsius. If your cylinder has no tempering valve, a plumber can install one.

Other safety precautions

Tape securely over electric switches for the fridge and deep freeze. Have a short flex on the electric kettle and take care where the cord for the iron dangles. Put it away after use.

Hide matches and ban cigarette lighters. If you can't persuade your charge to stop smoking, light their cigarettes yourself, and install a smoke alarm just outside the kitchen.

Use tight rubber bands to join cupboard doors where cleaning fluids and solvents are kept.

Messes and mopping up

Be prepared to buy special plates, cups and cutlery as eating skills slip. Build up a supply of old towels and kitchen bench cloths, and other large and small rags and sponges for mopping up spills.

The bathroom
Redecorating

A lot of future time may be spent in your bathroom. You may make your life easier by having it remodelled.

> One woman carer had the whole bathroom converted to a wet area. The shower box was taken out, a non-slip tile floor installed with a slope to a drainage hole, and everything brightened up. Her husband had space to wash himself all over more easily, and she could help if necessary.
>
> Another carer removed only the bath, because the shower was over it. A small wet area was put in, with tiles sloping down slightly to the ex-bath plughole.

If you are going to redo your bathroom, it is wise for safety's sake to have slip-resistant flooring, as wet tiles or wooden floors can cause awful tumbles. Have several easily washed, non-skid bath and toilet mats available, along with a rubber mat in the shower, and mop up any puddles immediately to prevent falls.

You could also consider installing taps that stop flowing after a limited time, or you can simply hide plugs to baths and basins, to avoid floods. A lever-operated water-mixer is easier to handle than individual tap knobs, and a hand-held spray attachment on a flexible hose is more practical than a fixed shower-head. Your shower can probably be adapted to this.

Have plenty of storage shelves or cupboards built above waist level, so that no one has to bend down for soap, towels and so on.

Access to rooms and equipment

For safety, have no locks on the bathroom and toilet doors, but keep a lock on the medicine cupboard. Electrical equipment – hairdryers, razors, and so on – should be in another room or out of sight and reach to avoid possible electric shocks. Plastic containers are more sensible than glass.

First aid kit

Your well-stocked first aid kit should include:
- assorted sterile gauze dressings (soaked in ointment so they won't stick to wounds) and ready-to-use sticking plasters in different sizes
- steri-strips, to pull wounds together
- crêpe and gauze bandages; safety pins or a roll of sticking plaster to hold them
- a continuous fabric dressing strip to cut to size for larger abrasions
- antiseptic/anaesthetic cream, for minor burns and abrasions
- cotton wool
- small, sharp medical scissors.

Mobility and stability

Consider adding a bathroom stool, the same height as the side of the bath, to make getting in and out of the bath easier, and to sit on in the shower or when cleaning teeth. Your occupational therapist can arrange for you to be supplied with other bathroom aids; often these are free.

It is almost standard, these days, to have a handle on the far wall above the bath. To make getting in and out easier, have another handle installed on the near side of the bath. You could also have handrails on two, or even three, sides in the shower box to give your charge something to hang on to instead of grabbing you or the curtains.

Strengthened shower curtain rails are good, in case your charge loses balance and grabs them. Consider also a wheelchair for showering, and a shower door that opens outwards. This makes helping much easier, though old habits may die hard.

> Owen, still showering himself, was dangerously unsteady getting around their inward-opening shower door, and it was almost impossible for Pauline to reach around it to help him wash his hair, so their occupational therapist had it changed to open outwards.
>
> The morning after this was done Pauline heard mighty clanging sounds in the bathroom, then Owen appeared in the kitchen naked, and told her he couldn't get into the shower. Puzzled, she went to investigate, and was dismayed and impressed in equal amounts by Owen's lack of understanding and his brute strength. He had managed to push the now outward-swinging door inwards, past the new door jamb made to hold it closed.

The bedroom
Covers and curtains

Choose plain fabrics. Patterns can confuse and, in some cases, cause hallucinations. Make sure the person you are looking after stays warm. Light duvets are better than heavier blankets; but, if they prefer blankets, don't change. Blankets can be a bit restrictive but are easier to tuck in to stay snug. Where duvets are used, carers sometimes find inventive ways to keep the bedding in place:

> Pamela was a restless sleeper and her bedding often slipped onto the floor. Peter eventually tied the top corner of her duvet to the end of the tape holding her electric blanket on the mattress. He finished it with a double bow, so it could not be pulled undone – not foolproof, but the best he could do.

◆

> Another carer sewed long tapes (which they passed under the mattress) to one side of the duvet, and shorter tapes on the other side. They attached clips (like those on children's pushchairs or car seats) to each tape end. When the person with dementia was

settled into bed, they clicked the clips together and pulled them firm. Their 'friend' could wriggle around all night without getting uncovered, but had to be released for the toilet.

Turning over in bed

Silk pyjamas will make turning over in bed easier for your charge. Avoid silk sheets, however: they make the bedding fall off too easily.

If they need help in turning, before they get into bed fold a sheet in three lengthways, then put it across the bed, where their bottom will be, leaving the sheet ends hanging down at the sides. When they want to turn over:
1. Fold back their bedclothes.
2. Pull the sheet by one end to one side and upwards (brace your feet on the mattress if necessary) so your charge is rolled and turned in the direction they wish to face.
3. Holding both ends of the sheet so your charge can't roll back again, pull your charge back into the middle of the bed and then put the sheet edges down both sides of the bed again, ready for the next 'turn'.

If your charge is incontinent, place a non-crackly plastic strip in the folded sheet.

Getting out of bed

People with dementia may become eligible for a hospital-supplied adjustable bed if they are assessed as needing one or have had a spell in hospital. These beds have controls to raise their feet higher than their head, or raise the person to a sitting position. From here you can help your charge to stand by moving their legs over to the side of the bed and down, and putting their feet onto the floor. A sturdy metal bedside table, complete with grab rail, can help your charge with this manoeuvre. Such a bed has adjustable rails on the sides, if required, to prevent the person from falling out.

Other bed-related equipment

Your occupational therapist may be able to supply other equipment.

For a single bed, a high, rounded metal handle at waist level on each side is useful. Attached to wooden boards that slip under the mattress, they provide a useful grip to help your charge turn. For a double bed, use one handle attached to a board under their side.

A 'monkey bar' is a curved bar that has a handle on a chain dangling above your charge's head. The person in bed can reach up and use it to change position, or pull themselves up to a sitting position. It is cumbersome but useful.

An electric air mattress prevents discomfort and bedsores by letting air flow continually but irregularly through pockets in its surface. This means that pressure points are never held too long. Another way to prevent bedsores is by using 'egg carton' mattress pads.

Calling the carer

If you don't sleep in the same bed or room you will need your charge to use a bell, to let you know when they want to get up. If they can't use a bell, set up a bedroom monitor; buy the type used for listening to babies.

If they refuse to go to bed, don't fuss. Let them sleep on a couch, in a recliner, or sit in an armchair – wherever they are happy.

Six-point checklist for night-time

1. Check the stove is off at the wall and remove element knobs.
2. Turn off and remove electric plugs from sockets, especially heaters.
3. Leave lights on in the kitchen (for snacking) and toilet; you will find mini-fluorescent bulbs are economical.
4. Activate child-proof door locks (see Chapter 22: Wandering).
5. Put away car keys.
6. Make sure the gate is across the top of any interior stairway.

Wheelchairs

If you eventually need a wheelchair for your charge, don't get one they can propel themselves. They can get into all sorts of trouble!

The best wheelchair should be light enough for you to put in your car on your own. See that its back stands higher than the occupant's head, to prevent pressure on their neck. It should also have a comfortable seat, and shoulder belts that can be put on lightly, to prevent the person with dementia from slipping out if they are rigid.

Use the wheelchair for no more than three hours a day, preferably wheeling it to different places for a change of scene. A wheelchair helps prevent bedsores later, if your charge enters hospital care.

Often a nearby pharmacist has wheelchairs for temporary hire. Try different ones before you buy.

People who want to continue living alone

You would be wise to alert neighbours to your charge's condition (although it would be unfair to depend on them) and adopt other precautions in this chapter. Realise, however, that there will be ongoing challenges.

> Martha had vascular dementia, but she also had a powerful personality and refused to move out of her own home. Valerie, her dutiful daughter, lived three streets away and engaged helpers to come in daily. They helped Martha shower and dress, prepared her lunch and dinner, and took her and her beloved Pekinese dog for a short walk.
>
> Martha refused to have anyone stay overnight; but if her Pekinese started yapping she would wake up terrified and phone her daughter to deal with 'the intruders'. This happened so often that Valerie, exhausted, finally refused to come. 'If you don't come, Valerie, I'll have to ring the police,' Martha threatened, and she did – so often that the police eventually phoned Valerie and complained.

Situations like this are fairly common. Each family has to work out its own ways to share the responsibilities. If unpleasantness erupts because they can't come to any agreement, a round-table discussion with another person or a counsellor can help solve differences.

Where to from here

✦ Chapter 6: Becoming a Carer, especially 'Events calendar tips'
✦ Chapter 7: Dealing with Health Professionals, especially 'Other help from the health industry'

- Chapter 11: Independence and Safety
- Chapter 19: Eating and Drinking
- Chapter 20: Showering and Dressing
- Chapter 21: Toileting
- Chapter 22: Wandering

Chapter 9

Managing Difficult Behaviour

Everyone with dementia has their own personal pathway. Your charge may retain many normal functions for years to come – or they may not. There are many common behaviours, however, and this chapter deals with some of them.

Fact and fantasy

Your charge may present fact and fantasy as equally real, and talk unbelievable nonsense about themselves. It's like children coming up with whopping stories, which they tend to do, once they can talk well enough to express their imagination.

Trevor swore he'd taken his pills – when he obviously hadn't.

♦

Ralph said he hadn't broken the crystal jug that Josie found in the rubbish bin when she came home.

♦

Carol said she hadn't touched her passport. It was found later tucked under her mattress.

Carol's action is a commonly experienced example of 'hiding' things, or putting them in outlandish places. She probably thought she was putting her passport somewhere safe.

Sometimes stories from television, the radio and books get jumbled up and become part of a person's own life experiences. Other times, lying may be a way of escaping from a dull daily environment, or of eliciting sympathy, or of getting support or avoiding trouble. The most likely reason for 'making things up', however, is that your charge has simply forgotten. It doesn't help to protest when you detect this, or to accuse them of anything. If they've always lied, you won't change them now; and if they've previously been truthful, this lying is the result of their condition.

Accept almost everything. Try not to be fazed. Don't argue for reality. And don't be too uptight about 'fudging' the truth yourself. Your charge will probably not remember what you said, and it may help you to manage a sticky situation.

> The leader of a carers' support group suggested that one new member, who had spent months coping with his wife on his own, 'Take it calmly and go along with whatever is on the menu.' He found that following this advice – accepting his wife as he found her rather than trying constantly to correct her – removed much of his daily strain.

You can also fudge it if a person with dementia wants to see someone who has died. Simply talk about the person, help find their photo in an album, or say they will be around later.

Another option is to engage in more elaborate play-acting:
> Kirsten's agitated mother wanted to be in touch with her very old friend, who had died 20 years previously. Kirsten phoned her sister and arranged for her to pretend to be that old friend. She gave the phone to her mother and a long phone conversation ensued, from which their mother gained much satisfaction.

◆

> When a person with dementia wanted to speak with their parents (who were dead), the carer pretended to phone them and have an animated conversation, asking about what they – Mum and Dad – had been doing that day. The carer went on to discuss gardening, what was being cooked, having friends in, doing the washing, shopping, feeding the dog … then turned around to say that Mum and Dad apologised for being too tired to talk any more, but 'I can tell you their news.' Afterwards, talking about the 'news' and the past gave the person with dementia some contentment.

Sometimes there's no need to sidestep or to create a story, as your charge doesn't absorb the truth or see that the situation or person has anything to do with them.

> While driving to the hospital where her father lay dying after a massive coronary, a daughter warned her mother that he might not be alive when they reached him. The man had devotedly looked after his wife, who had Alzheimer's, for several years – yet only a momentary flicker of emotion came over the woman's face before she said brightly, 'Just look at that enormous bus!'
>
> On the day of her husband's funeral, people at the wake made an extra fuss of her. As she left, she exclaimed, 'I've had such a happy day!'

Losing track of people

If someone appears in your charge's life for a short time and is quickly forgotten, you will probably be unruffled. When you and your charge have been close for years and they suddenly have no idea who you are, it's another story. Though you know it's the dementia talking, you may feel the need to go away and shed some tears. Don't be hard on yourself – or them – about the incident.

> It was their wedding anniversary. They'd got dressed up in their best clothes and were waiting to go out with the family, when Jeffrey turned to Janine and said, 'I know it's my wedding anniversary, but I can't remember who I married. Can you tell me?'

One common mistake with familiar figures of the 'here and now' is to misidentify them as people from long ago.

> One man began calling his daughter 'Mother'. Rather than being hurt that he didn't recognise her for who she was, the daughter was glad that he associated her with his much-loved mother.

Losing track of time

Don't argue if your charge says, 'Why do you go away and leave me all day?' when you have been gone only five minutes. Say, 'Oh, you do miss me!' or 'You feel lonely when I'm not there.'

A mother phoned from her long-term care residence: 'Do you know where to pick me up tomorrow?' she asked.

'Yes, Mum, I know where you are,' her daughter replied.

'I'm here at my job, you know?' the older woman said. 'I want to come home.'

'Yes, I know where you are, Mum,' her daughter reassured her.

'I'll be there at the right time.'

The daughter was wise to avoid argument about either 'my job', or coming home. Argument would only have distressed her mother, who by the next day would probably have forgotten their 'arrangement'.

People with dementia don't always forget the arrangements they have with carers, however, even if they no longer have an accurate sense of time.

'Alison, Alison, where are you?' Bruce's voice, hoarse from Lewy body dementia, came down the phone-line to his wife. 'I've been waiting for you to come all day.'

It was 1.50 pm. She had already visited him earlier, because she had an important meeting elsewhere at their usual afternoon time. However, upset by his call, she went back to the hospital after her meeting finished at 4.15 pm. Bruce was sitting in a wheelchair outside the hospital office.

'He wanted to see you so much,' said the matron, Mary, who had called Alison's number for him. 'I let him stay all afternoon after I heard him speak to you. He wouldn't be moved.'

Non-responsive times

At times the person you are caring for may be quite unresponsive. If they seem calm and contented there is no reason to disturb them, but be aware and near in case they need you. But if you sense unhappiness – for instance, if they sit frowning and slumped, head hanging, mouth turned down – you may need to take some action.

If they accept being touched, give them hugs or gentle pats, put your arm around their shoulder, stroke their hair or kiss their cheek or the back of their neck. Alternatively tuck a rug around them and find them a foot stool, sit close and hold their hand, or lie with your arms around them in bed. If there is a rocking chair in the house, they may love it if you sit rocking with them cuddled on your lap. Of course, if they don't like being touched, all that might produce much worse temper!

Another way you may be able to turn these bad or sad moods around is with their life book. Sit with them, turn pages and talk about days past, avoiding questions. Instead say: 'Tell me about when you...' or 'Tell me what you did when...' They can enjoy reminiscing about the old days again and again, and you may sometimes be surprised by new things they mention. There can be much behind those often mask-like faces.

If you suspect definite depression, seek treatment quickly from your doctor.

Sundowning or twilighting

These behaviours, mainly agitation, confusion and restlessness, are common in people with dementia and usually begin in the late afternoon. They sometimes continue throughout the night, with you and your charge completely worn out the next day.

Examples include bursting into the room and yelling, 'Come on, we've got to start packing or we'll miss the train!' ('Oh, no,' you groan to yourself) or 'Time for all you fellas to get up. You've got to be at footie practice.' (They think the children, who are all now married, are still at home and have to be shaken out of bed, even though it's 4.30 pm.)

Because you are tired, depressed and frustrated, the inclination is to yell back at them not to be silly: there is no one else in the house, the children are all married, it's late in the afternoon – and then you remember. Your reaction is understandable and forgivable, but you may still feel guilty.

Ways of coping

Sedatives are not the answer to sundowning, as they could lead to more unsteadiness and depression. Avoid alcohol, too. Apart from the fact that it doesn't mix well with most medications, it can increase anxiety and confusion.

Limit drinks containing caffeine (coffee, energy drinks, cola, chocolate) to mornings only. Taper off activities as evening comes, just as you would with a young child.

Spend time outside, or sit inside near natural light. Exposure to sunlight helps set the body's internal clock and may also improve your charge's mood.

Regular times for going to bed and getting up are important: try to keep them the same as when your charge had a regular working day. If they sleep late in the mornings, wake them tactfully. Limit daytime sleeps, too. This is difficult with someone who spends much of the day sitting and dozing; but try to make real rests not too late in the day, and taken on a couch or reclining chair, rather than on their bed. Keep their bed for night-time.

Have on-the-spot quiet distractions handy: a craft activity, something for them to hold, feel or fiddle with, or go for an easy walk. Afternoon exercise will help ensure they are tired by evening.

Another strategy is to select peaceful radio or television programmes. Collect a series of DVDs they find absorbing on favourite cooking or sports programmes, animal features or war films. They will watch them over and over and never remember, but feel relaxed because they seem familiar. Be sure you relax yourself, so you're better prepared in case sundowning still erupts.

As dusk falls, turn on lots of lights to prevent any confusing shadows, and close blinds or curtains against the dark. Have minimal noise, disorder and people about.

Sitting in a rocking chair can be soothing, as can listening to much-loved music and talking about the memories it brings up.

Before bedtime a gentle backrub might relax them (see Chapter 15: Maintaining Health, 'Natural therapies'). Alternatively try a warm bath, a light snack and a milky drink, but make sure they don't have too much fluid. Have that warm milk or herbal tea available for the middle of the night as well.

Routine, routine, routine: this will help to comfort them and produce nice dreams.

Mood swings

Dementia produces unexpected changes in your charge's moods and reactions as social skills dissolve. Have plans for dealing with such occasions.

> Margot had always been a quiet woman, but she became increasingly agitated and difficult to soothe as her Alzheimer's progressed. Her feelings hung out wherever she happened to be, and she sometimes even gate-crashed meetings her husband was involved in.
>
> He knew she could be like this for up to two hours, so would sit her down beside him without embarrassment, put his arms around her and stroke her forehead and carry on. Other times on their own, he talked quietly to her, or read to her, or walked her around, or sang to her – and she would sometimes join in. These were his strategies to make her agitation pass more quickly.

You may know your charge well enough to know what is soothing or distracting enough: perhaps it will mean holding a familiar object or hearing a favourite song.

If you don't yet know what will work, you are likely to learn from experience very soon!

Antisocial behaviour

Your charge may embarrass you greatly at times. Sexual behaviour in public or in company is not uncommon, and can be particularly awkward. Even if the initiator is unselfconscious because of their dementia, the recipients may feel differently.

> Ryan would touch women's breasts when he and his wife were out at social gatherings.
>
> ◆
>
> When Esther and Aaron met their lawyer to talk family trust business, she put her arm round the lawyer's waist and tried to fondle his crotch.

They don't have to be explicitly sexual or intentionally intimidating for those around them to feel uncomfortable.

Arnold wandered into the female patients' bedrooms and dressed up in their clothes. They were frightened, although he didn't threaten them in any way.

◆

A man's loud voice could occasionally be heard upstairs, shortly after Bruce moved into his new, full-time care home. One morning the man himself appeared downstairs. He was sixtyish, almost two metres tall, very well-built and stark naked. He laughed loudly, raised both arms in the air and bellowed, 'Good morning to you all,' and came and sat down in an armchair opposite Bruce's wife Alison.

She felt embarrassed and discomfited. She murmured, 'Good morning,' and turned back to Bruce.

A nurse arrived quickly and spoke respectfully to the man: 'Well, Mr ____, you're out of your rented space down here, aren't you? Please follow me back upstairs.' She turned and led the way, and he meekly got up and followed her.

In the cases above, experienced staff were responsible for finding a solution. But you may be the only 'staff' on hand when your charge does something like this. If so, and if you need to remove them from the situation, it is important that you avoid making a fuss.

Explain as calmly as possible to the people on the receiving end that dementia is in the driving seat, and that your charge is not to blame. Your Alzheimer's organisation may have an explanatory card that carers can show to strangers who become involved.

Is it really so bad?

The stigma associated with dementia probably arises because of strange remarks, imagined violence, or 'unacceptable' behaviour by some people with dementia. Nudity, grossly rude talk and so on can cause uneasy reactions from onlookers.

Consider, though, that near-nudity is to be seen at public beaches and swimming pools, as well as in films, theatres, cabarets and strip clubs. Grossly rude behaviour occurs sometimes in shops, restaurants and even in one's own home; and our society is full of people getting away with all sorts of illegal, licentious or immoral sexual actions. These are done by people with full mental faculties and in responsible jobs.

Where to from here
+ Chapter 11: Independence and Safety
+ Chapter 12: Feelings
+ Chapter 13: Communication
+ Chapter 14: Intimacy, Love and Sex
+ Chapter 21: Toileting
+ Chapter 22: Wandering
+ Chapter 23: Hallucinations, Delusions and Delirium
+ Chapter 24: Aggression

Chapter 10

Wider Support and Self-care

How the wider family can help

Families can be crucial in determining the quality of life for a person with dementia and their principal carer, for good or for ill.

Some family members respond negatively on hearing of a dementia diagnosis. They can be embarrassed and uncomfortable with the person with dementia, refuse to accept any responsibilities, even break off contact. Some may gossip to their friends; others may start underhand financial strategies.

Many will rally around, however, and there is a wide range of ways they can make life easier for you and the person you are looking after by:

- reading extensively about the dementia and sharing the information with everyone
- learning to cope practically with all facets of the disease
- noticing new symptoms and letting you know
- coordinating their own support services – telephone networking, visiting schedule, and so on
- involving family members who live in another area
- sharing the physical aspects of keeping your person with dementia as occupied and content as possible
- making new suggestions for coping
- suggesting and sharing in plans for your charge's care if they choose to live with a professional carer, or even alone in their own home
- helping with budgeting to cover financial contingencies.

Sensitivity

Sometimes the best way people can help is by being sensitive – by noticing non-verbal cues and acting on them, in the best interests of the person with dementia and their carer.

> Earl sat hunched up in his chair. Linda, his elder daughter, had arrived to visit him during his respite care, and Gillian, his younger daughter, turned up at the same time with her three little children. They all made a lot of noise with their animated chatter. Earl's eyes darted from person to person, his hands began shaking and he became agitated. Too many people! Linda raised her eyebrows at Gillian who understood, said goodbye quickly to her father, and took her mob away.
> 'Who were those awful people?' Earl asked.
> 'That was Gillian, your daughter, and your grandchildren,' replied Linda.
> 'I've never seen them before in my life,' Earl said peevishly.

Balancing support and 'labour'

Family members should ideally talk first to the principal carer about their possible role. The best thing the family can do is be kind and patient, instead of tiring themselves trying to help with the physical work of caring. Some may do lots of wearying tasks and end up full of resentment towards both the carer and the person with dementia.

They may do this 'helping' to reduce your costs, not knowing about the free support which is available. Their emotional support is more important than their practical support, although, of course, some of that is needed as well.

From a distance

If you are a relative who lives far away, but still wish to have input, you can most usefully offer a listening, sympathetic ear for the caregiver on the spot – especially if they live in an isolated place. Encourage them to let off steam to you via phone, email or text; but don't offer advice unless they ask you for it. Laugh with them as well as empathising at their horror stories, even if they shock you.

Tips for 'distance caring'
- Phone regularly.
- Send an occasional bunch of flowers or a gift basket to show how much you value the role they have taken on.
- Give petrol vouchers or something to acknowledge the additional travel involved in caregiving (seeing doctors and so on), or the expense of long-distance phone calls.
- Arrange to spend time with the person with dementia and give their carer a break whenever you travel to visit them.
- Make sure the carer gets regular appropriate breaks, especially at Christmas or school holiday times, perhaps by taking over for a week or two a year.
- Send notes/letters/photographs telling current news, or parcels, to the person with dementia.
- Contribute financially.

Self-care
Many caregivers offer themselves up as sacrifices on the altar of duty. But to do the job effectively and regularly, you need to care for yourself as well as the person you are looking after.

After a period as caregiver
One way to work out whether you are coping is to consider whether you:
- feel that whatever you do is not enough
- have sudden mood changes and difficulty making decisions
- need alcohol, pills or drugs to see you through
- find it hard to complete routine tasks
- feel overwhelmed and bewildered
- get angry with yourself or your charge
- find it becoming increasingly difficult to face each day
- struggle with weight loss/gain, sleeplessness, headaches, or frequent colds/infections
- feel your relationships with others are deteriorating
- think about suicide.

If you identify with some of these statements you could well be overloaded and could be heading for depression. It is important that you reach out to somebody you trust and seek medical help.

The Carer's Code

You, your charge and everybody around you will benefit if you read the Carer's Code below, take note, and promise to follow the Code. It applies to any caregiver, not only those looking after dementia patients.

As a caregiver, I must remember to do the following:
1. Take good care of myself and recognise my limits, without feeling I am failing to measure up. This is not selfish. It will enable me to take better care of my charge.
2. Ask for help whenever I think I need it, even though my charge may object.
3. Keep up my own interests and activities, while doing everything that I reasonably can for my charge, just as I would if they were healthy.
4. Realise it is normal to feel anger or depression occasionally, and to express these and other difficult feelings to a support group.
5. Reject any attempts by my charge to manipulate me (consciously or subconsciously) through their anger, guilt, self-pity or depression.
6. Feel entitled to receive consideration – affection, acceptance, forgiveness – for what I do, as long as I am offering these qualities. I must make sure that my charge and I give each other hugs, and laugh often.
7. Take pride in what I am accomplishing, including the effort and courage it sometimes takes to cope.
8. Preserve my individuality and right to live my own life in preparation for the time when my charge will need less of my care. I must keep in touch with my friends.
9. Have a support group, and expect to be supported as a caregiver by medical staff and others, just as my charge is. If this is not the case, I must go to another doctor.
10. Feel content with myself and what I am doing, even without direct feedback, acknowledgement or praise.

11. Imagine realistic goals and write them down.
12. Follow all the above. It is easy to give advice, but very difficult to apply it to myself. (See 1 and 3 above.)

Time out

You may find that not everybody in your life approves of these steps. Your charge may, or may not, accept that you are sometimes off duty and off site. Others who don't understand the demands of the job may look askance. But self-care is essential, and so is taking time out. You may need to be creative or insistent about this.

> Marcus was deteriorating, and his partner and carer, Sheena, just had to have a break. When he was due for his first respite care, Marcus refused to go anywhere, and said that if she wanted a break, she'd have to take herself off. This is what Sheena did, though she had to be resourceful in finding a solution to Marcus's care.
>
> Sheena knew there would be a major bust-up if she insisted that Marcus went to a 'home', so she arranged to pay for help to come in to look after him each day, and for a couple who lived not far away to cook the evening meal and sleep in the spare room for a week.
>
> She booked herself into a motel by a local beach, chose a pile of good books and set off with her bathing suit, sun hat, a few clothes and a light heart. Some of her friends applauded her wisdom, others criticised her severely, but her family was very supportive.

Support groups

Support groups are small, and in many cases meetings are arranged monthly by support staff of agencies promoting the interests of people living with dementia – either those with the condition or their carers. Meetings can be very informal, member-driven gatherings held during a morning tea or lunch break and lasting 60–90 minutes. A support person may be present to facilitate the conversation and answer any questions (not to lecture).

Support groups introduce you to other people in similar situations and help you feel you are not alone. They can also help you learn more about what assistance is available and find out how others cope with their different situations. From this you can work out your own ways, thus lessening your stresses.

> Helen and Alison met at a support group lunch. Helen exclaimed when she heard how little help Alison had with her husband's care. She listed the assistance she herself was receiving: 'Someone to shower and dress Don every morning, people coming in during the week so I can get out more, and he's going into respite care for two weeks every eight weeks.'
>
> Alison was silent. She couldn't take all that in immediately, but she sensed that she should. 'Tell me that again slowly,' she said. 'I'd be a better carer if…'
>
> She learned so much at that first lunch she could hardly wait for the next one.

Not everyone joins support groups easily. You may think you are happier battling along on your own.

> Sally was devastated when her Lionel was diagnosed with dementia, but she fronted up strongly. She had held responsible jobs, and reckoned she knew how to care for him. She spurned help she was offered, and became more and more exhausted.
>
> When Lionel finally died, Sally gradually rejoined the community. She now heard how some carers and their charges got together in groups, and at other times carers met to share their experiences, coping strategies and news about day-care facilities and respite care.
>
> Sally wondered whether she and Lionel had been right to keep to themselves. She had been safeguarding his dignity, she admitted afterwards: she couldn't bear anyone to see her spruce, handsome husband become a shambling wreck.

Perhaps you have been to one meeting and felt on the outer, or that the chemistry was not right. Do try again – even with one, two or three different support groups – before you decide against it.

Quick recuperation for carers

Lie on your back on the floor for five minutes with your head on a low cushion and your lower legs resting at right angles on a sofa or chair. This is a yoga resting position. You may think you look ridiculous, but five minutes like this is equivalent to much more time on your bed, and you can do it while keeping an eye on your charge. It may give them a laugh, too. You might read the newspaper or a book at the same time, holding it above your head, but you will probably find your eyes close and you have a short, refreshing nap.

Where to from here

✦ Chapter 4: Dealing with the News
✦ Chapter 12: Feelings
✦ Chapter 13: Communication
✦ Chapter 26: Moving into Full-time Care, especially 'When they don't speak'

Part Three

Balancing Acts

Chapter 11

Independence and Safety

A lifetime of experience

When someone in your life is diagnosed with dementia, the door doesn't instantly clang shut on every bit of wisdom that they have accumulated over their life.

> Phillip scuffed shoes when he walked, he dribbled, his nose ran, his face had no expression and he couldn't concentrate. Sylvia could hardly hear him speak and he got lost driving to his son's place; but when he began getting lost in his own home she realised she had been avoiding the truth.
>
> Dementia was diagnosed. 'But he's not crazy,' Sylvia said. 'He's not at all what I thought a "demented" person would be like. He's still my Phillip.'
>
> Her husband was prescribed Exelon (rivastigmine), with a warning it might make him feel sick. He retorted that the price made him feel sick, and refused to take it. 'That's what the doctors told me,' Sylvia mused. 'He might have dementia, but he'll still have his wits about him!'

A person with dementia has made a similar point:

> We, and the people like us, will have to develop new ways to cope with the new ways our brains are operating. Life will go on differently and at a reducing speed, but we will still be the people we were, with our lifetime of experience, knowledge and wisdom – we will just be slower and slower accessing them.

Chapter 11

A sense of independence

Retaining a sense of independence will remain important for the person with dementia for a long time. Increasingly, you and others will need to make decisions for them, but be careful about taking over when you don't need to.

Try to balance any joint decision-making by letting them decide things themselves for as long as possible. Don't be surprised when you find them more than capable.

> Donald had lost most of his teeth, and his doctor said he needed a denture. His wife, Helen, doubted he could manage it, given his dementia, but had a gut feeling that Donald had to decide.
>
> They went to the hospital's free dental service for the extraction of his remaining top teeth, but Donald stopped the dentist's hand holding the hypodermic needle as it came near. 'Is this really necessary?' he asked.
>
> 'Well, it's over to you, Donald,' replied the white-masked dental surgeon.
>
> Donald pondered, then said, 'Well, I don't want to go ahead. I think I will say no.'
>
> 'Okay, young fellow,' the dentist murmured, 'if you say no, no it is.'
>
> Helen said nothing, and three years later Donald could still chew a mouthful with the one remaining top tooth – and swallow the result.

Do you really need to say 'no'?

Sometimes the person you are looking after will exercise poor judgement, but so does every human being. Rather than immediately and conclusively saying 'no' to your charge, you may need to weigh up whether the issue under discussion really matters more than their happiness at this moment.

> Ann, who always included Reg in household goings-on, told him they had enough 'reward' points for a bonus purchase. Although he had difficulty reading, Reg browsed through the catalogue. 'This is what we need,' he said, pointing to an illustration of an electric hedge clipper.

It would be too much for Reg's wasting muscles and his dodderiness, Ann realised, but he kept on and on. Rather than leave him out of their decision-making, she ordered the hedge clipper.

Ann knew her husband well enough to predict that, once the appliance was in his hands, he would quickly recognise his inability to manage it. He did, and as bonus purchases couldn't be returned, it was sent to their daughter's home. 'We can borrow it when we need it, darling,' Ann soothed Reg, who was very disappointed.

One woman with dementia praised her husband for supporting her activity and independence, and another person urged other carers to do the same:

> My husband is my bulwark. The best thing about him is that he is willing to let me do as much as I can by myself. He does not hover over me and tell me I can't do things. Instead, he offers support and encouragement. I never feel inadequate when he's around.

◆

> We need time and space to try things. Keep us doing as much as possible. Don't take over! Let us make mistakes or fail, but don't make us feel we are failures. Help us not to give up. Help us find new ways to cope.

Wanting to participate

Dementia reduces people's ability to function at a level previously enjoyed, or to define themselves by responsible positions that they hold at work or at home. It is crucial that those around them are sensitive to how this feels.

> One person with dementia said, in frustration, 'People ask me how I'm spending my time – I'm not earning anything!' Another commented, 'I feel like I'm left out on the side of the road … like I don't have anything to do any more.'

When the ability to make decisions is much reduced, there is still a desire to participate in life. One way to do this is by letting them help out rather than sidelining them, as this carer discovered:

> At first when we went on picnics or had family dinners I tended to say, 'You just relax and enjoy yourself,' because for most of

us relaxing is a luxury. But I stopped when I realised she felt that helping gave her status and pleasure – but only for simple tasks.

Of course, you can be too insistent about keeping up activity levels, so this is another balancing act for carers. Many people with dementia want to be asked first whether they want to do something before being rushed into it.

No longer able to manage

At various points along the dementia path, your charge needs to give up activities they have taken for granted. This is especially difficult if they won't accept that they can no longer manage them.

Living alone

Living alone, including cooking simple meals, is one area of sensitivity. One compromise is to accommodate the person with dementia in a separate flat within the family home, though eventually that also becomes too hard for all concerned.

> Petra's mother, who had multi-infarct dementia as the result of several strokes, had chosen to live alone in a little cottage at the end of Petra's garden. She rang late one night, sounding confused and frightened. She couldn't remember where her bedroom was. Petra had to go and tuck her up.
>
> Another time, her mother rang and screamed that she was on fire. Petra dashed over and found her mother standing in her bedroom looking vacant. 'Oh, I really thought I was on fire,' she gasped, wrapping her dressing gown more tightly around herself.

When safety is paramount, you may need to insist that the person with dementia no longer live on their own. Perhaps you can put the responsibility elsewhere by saying that the fire brigade has informed you that your charge may no longer use the stove, or have access to cigarettes and matches, or something similar.

Managing money

At another point, the person you are caring for will no longer be sensible with money. Keep as little cash in the house as possible, but give them a small-denomination banknote or a number of coins to carry around if they wish. Don't give them a number of notes, because they may be careless with them or others may take advantage of them.

Getting out and about

Early on, they may still be driving simple routes, but their increasing physical limitations may make it difficult to park the car and reach the proper floor at the hospital, dentist or other venue. They may not be able to manage the steps into public transport.

When this stage is reached, know that some taxi companies offer reduced fares to anyone assessed by Parkinson's, Alzheimer's or other societies as needing help. Always show the driver the mobility concession card before the start of the trip, and keep a generous collection of gold coins for your charge's pocket, to pay fares easily at their destination.

Also, obtain a disabled person's car-parking card, for when you are doing the driving. You may need your doctor's signature on the application form.

When driving is no longer safe

Dealing with your charge's driving as it deteriorates can be one of the most puzzling and difficult exercises for you as carer. Although it is obvious to people around them that they should not be driving, they are sublimely unaware of the danger, not only to themselves but to everyone on the roads around them.

> By nature William was courteous, but as a driver he was always too fast and too close to the car in front. He would never let June, his wife, take the wheel when they travelled together, and she couldn't stand up to him – not even when he developed Parkinson's disease, nor when dementia began creeping in.
>
> One Friday they set off to spend a weekend with friends. William sped along at 120–140 kph and June dozed uneasily. Suddenly she was woken by the wheels skittering over gravel and the car bumping violently. Brambles and a farm fence loomed as William braked hard and spun the wheel. The car skidded, turned

towards the safety of rough grass beside the road and, moments later, was gliding back on the asphalt. June's heart was pumping madly. 'I must have fallen asleep for a moment,' William muttered, staring grimly straight ahead.

'Will!' June exclaimed. 'What would've happened if there'd been the usual ditch – a lamppost – a tree?' They travelled on at 90 kph in troubled silence.

Three ways to prevent driving

If the person you are looking after is not safe to drive but may still try, you could try the following:
1. Hide the car keys.
2. Use a removable steering lock and hide the key.
3. Pull the driver's seat forward against the steering wheel.

If they can't overcome these measures, they should not be driving.

Taking a test

Someone with dementia is five times more likely to have an accident than those of similar age without dementia. Your insurer must be told about your charge's medical diagnosis, or the company will not pay out if they have an accident. Perhaps this sobering news will prompt some people to give up driving. If not, there is another way.

June finally made an appointment to see their doctor alone, to ask him if he could stop William from driving. Will had driven through red lights, dented his car all over from minor collisions, and been stopped by a traffic officer when he was weaving between lanes without signalling. Finding only a doddery old man instead of the drunk driver he expected, the officer had let him go with a caution.

The doctor sighed when he heard this. 'If I advise William to stop driving, June, he'll never come to me again,' he said. 'Colleagues have told me this. It's incredibly difficult. He might kill someone, if not himself or you. The Automobile Association supports a place where drivers can go to be tested, but getting William to take the test is going to be the hard part.'

Independence and Safety

June finally wrote to his hospital specialist, who at their next appointment tactfully told William that with his medical condition he would not be covered by insurance … unless he took an AA test to prove his driving was okay.

Soon after, William crumpled his car badly and decided that he'd take the test and show everyone that he really was still fit to drive. He not only got lost on the way to the testing site, but he then became completely confused during the procedure. When the examiner told him he could no longer drive, William retorted, 'But you didn't even see me driving, and you tested me on a computer, and I don't even use a computer.'

'No,' replied the examiner, 'it may seem unfair to those who are not computer-literate, but these computers test reaction time, not computer skills. They are a completely fair initial measure of driving ability.'

'So how am I going to get home?' William had challenged, and was given permission to drive home for the last time. He was furious for the rest of his life.

Of comfort is the research confirming that it is cheaper to take taxis if you travel less than 5000 kilometres a year in your car. Of no comfort at all is the fact that people with dementia may find being stripped of their driving licence one of the most demeaning, horrible times in their lives. They may moan about it for years. Or they may become dedicated back-seat drivers:

Edgar flinched as Rosie, his wife, drove along the road. 'Hey, you were mighty lucky not to hit that car! Be more careful. You went far too close!' he barked.

Rosie slowed down and looked in her rear-vision mirror. 'What car, Edgar? There's nothing parked there.'

'I tell you, you missed it by inches!'

Rosie turned around and drove slowly past the way they had come, then did a U-turn and drove back again.

'Mmm,' said Edgar. 'It must've moved off. I'm sure there was a car there when we came past last time.'

He was having one of his Lewy body dementia hallucinations.

Where to from here
- Chapter 7: Dealing with Health Professionals
- Chapter 8: Adapting the Home Environment
- Chapter 9: Managing Difficult Behaviour
- Chapter 12: Feelings
- Chapter 13: Communication
- Chapter 22: Wandering
- Chapter 23: Hallucinations, Delusions and Delirium
- Chapter 25: Choosing Full-time Care, especially 'Use of restraints'

Chapter 12

Feelings

After a diagnosis of dementia you can have torrents of mixed feelings. Usually, we deal well enough with physically painful feelings: apply cold water to a burn, go to hospital with a broken leg, or to the doctor with an ulcer. Many of us, though, don't know what to do with the mental pain that we feel when, perhaps, someone is rude or dismissive or unfaithful. If we have been brought up to suppress our feelings (especially negative ones), the effect is like that of a clamp – stopping a natural, healing reaction.

Emotional self-control can be called for sometimes; but, overused, it can become ingrained, harm relationships with other people and ultimately affect your physical health, contributing perhaps to stomach ulcers, heart attacks or other health problems. If people reach out to you and invite you to be candid about your feelings only to have you cover up or change the subject, it may be a waste of a good opportunity and they may stop calling.

> People would ring up solicitously, asking how I was, or more often how the 'old fella' was. I always replied automatically, 'Oh, fine, thanks,' when in fact we were having a dreadful day. I was exhausted.

The woman quoted here is beginning to recognise how she is hiding her feelings. Ideally, she and you could (if you don't already):

- name your own feelings and practise ways of managing them constructively (see '"I" messages', below)
- identify what your charge is feeling, then talk to them about it (see 'Your charge's feelings', below).

By dealing with feelings, we help solve problems and avoid the corrosive effect of bottling them up.

Identifying your feelings

In the following passage, names of some feelings, all of them common, are in square brackets. Consider how often you identify them in yourself.

> A while ago you may have regarded yourself as independent [feeling free, self-sufficient] as a son or daughter, sibling, or partner. You had shrugged off the responsibilities [feeling liberated, unattached, privileged, relaxed] that you had carried when you were younger, or working, or were a parent with children at home. You were enjoying this freedom [feeling happy, contented, fortunate, thankful] and were planning [feeling anticipation, excitement, optimism] to make the most of it.
>
> You have been stunned [feeling inadequate, helpless, dazed, anxious] by the diagnosis of dementia – even though you may have had your suspicions [feeling fear, insecurity, uncertainty, uneasiness]. Your new obligations and ties as a 'principal carer' have left you crushed [feeling afraid, defenceless, horrified, impotent, blocked, disconcerted, upset, afflicted]. You may have concerns [feeling perplexed, confounded, threatened] about the life ahead. You sense [feeling forlorn, apprehensive] that you have lost your independence.

The bracketed words are some of more than 200 common feelings that can be listed in groups headed Mad, Sad, Bad, Glad, Scared. Expand your emotional vocabulary. It will be easier to name your emotions and those of the person you are looking after.

You can be upset by all sorts of things and in all sorts of ways. You can even be upset with the person you are looking after for becoming ill, and you may be shocked that you sometimes even wish they would die.

Guilt is something you can expect to feel often. It sometimes follows other emotions – you may feel guilty about things you discover you feel, such as critical of/fed up with/put upon by the person you look after – but that doesn't make the feeling less powerful. If you tell yourself guiltily that your feelings are wrong, when your charge is the one suffering, remind yourself that you are suffering as a result of their suffering, and that if you are feeling something, you are truly feeling it.

Other feelings that may become familiar include embarrassment and disbelief in the wake of some activity or accident.

> Frank suddenly wet his trousers and made a huge puddle on the
> doorstep of the motel unit.

Resentment is another common and understandable feeling in the face of repeated demands.

> If I am upstairs he will find excuses to keep me going up and down.
> Either he is going to faint, or he wants to go the toilet, or he can't
> get himself out of a chair – all quite valid reasons for calling me – so
> that I can't take chances by ignoring them.

Your charge's feelings

Your charge still has a personality. As dementia develops they may be more of what they previously were: if they were always dominant, they may become impossibly bossy; if they were meek, they may become impossibly self-effacing, vague or repetitive. Conversely, sometimes personality changes can occur and they become the opposite!

People with dementia are full of feelings and wishes, urges and hopes, like the rest of us. They, too, can sometimes find little joy in the present and see no jot of it in the future. Their feelings, though, may be locked away behind walls of increasing disabilities; they can less easily express them.

Their feelings may be different from yours, or have a different basis. They may feel the shame of their dementia label, the physical side-effects of drugs, and panic caused by the diagnosis.

Ways to deal with feelings

It may warm the cockles of their heart if you name feelings for them, especially if they have greater difficulty than you in doing this: 'Oh, you're [pleased, miserable, proud, resentful – or whatever] at the moment.' They may even take pleasure in telling you if you are wrong.

> Russell could neither read nor make sense of his old company's minutes (which they continued to send him). He was getting furious and wouldn't admit to himself how much he minded 'losing it'.
>
> Maisie expressed his frustration for him. 'It makes you so mad, Russell. It's so frustrating you can't do what you used to. Here, I'll read them to you. You like to know what's going on.'

Perhaps the person you are looking after is worried and going on about it. If, for instance, a grandchild staying with you has not come home on time, you could say: 'What a worry they are. Grandchildren! You wonder if they're okay.' Then you explain, 'He/she is staying at a friend's house tonight.'

If they become frustrated and unhappy with what they are doing, agree (with empathy) that life is not easy. Don't ask open questions; instead make positive statements. Say, 'Oh life's a bummer. These downers are really hard to take.' They may be comforted by your empathy, or stimulated into a denial that leads them to name their feelings more accurately.

Say something nice to them: 'Don't forget I love/am very fond of/like you so much.' Try distracting them with another activity. They can return to what they were doing later, if necessary. When their feelings get on top of them, you and they can achieve nothing.

If you both talk about being upset with the dementia dilemma, you can both feel a form of release, although you will be sharing it, of course, from different perspectives.

Loneliness
The person with dementia

Social contact is what makes us human beings; yet it is devilishly difficult to have social contact if you can't understand easily what people are saying and can't talk properly in reply.

> One doctor commented that he saw people ignoring people with dementia because their blank faces made them look as though they were not interested, but he knew they were.

Your charge may have a great sense of aloneness as they battle with their condition, or they may never want to go out because of their sense of inadequacy. Try to be empathetic. Let them talk about it.

Your own isolation

Be aware, too, that you can feel 'left out of things' as a result of your charge's lack of contact and your need to look after them. Friends go to films, or on trips; they have parties, talk about their grandchildren or gossip about latest goings-on. Life goes on without you, and you can imagine an unknown number of years of this. Gloom of one sort or another may develop, or you may shovel blame on to your charge and take it out on them by being irritable – or worse.

A carer's sense of isolation can be exacerbated by the changes in the person they look after. One daughter commented:

> My mother does not remember me or my father, who died many years ago. When I talk about earlier times – about pets and holidays, for instance – she looks blank. Since she's been diagnosed it's been awfully difficult. It is like living with a stranger, someone who keeps aloof and doesn't want to be touched. And she was so dear to me. If I try to hug her, she says, 'Don't be silly. Go away.'

If both of you are lonely, consider admitting to your charge that you feel as they do – and seek help from others.

> After having Parkinson's for four years Tanya gradually developed dementia. Along with this came some pitiful self-consciousness, especially in public, and she refused to go out, even with family and friends. Warren missed their mates and felt she was being unfair. He protested, and they argued a lot. They told all this to Tanya's doctor, who suggested counselling, but Tanya went only twice before refusing to go again. Warren continued, however, finding the sessions very useful; he later located a monthly online support group for people with similar problems. They quite quickly became new friends, and he could go out and do things with them.

Depression

Be aware that depression may creep up on you or (as with the emotions above) on the person you are caring for. It may show up in either of you as:
- loss of interest in usually enjoyed activities
- neglecting personal care

- ✦ feeling worthless, hopeless, sad and guilty
- ✦ having exaggerated, self-critical thoughts
- ✦ difficulty in concentrating or making decisions (perhaps you don't expect your charge to make decisions anyway)
- ✦ tearful episodes, agitation, worry, irritability, recklessness
- ✦ changes in eating or sleeping habits
- ✦ low energy, headache, digestive problems, aching body.

The sensations may be short-term, and a result of physical infection – so get them checked out. Alternatively this may be a developing long-term condition. Some unhappiness about their deteriorating condition is to be expected, but not dark despondency. Get a medical opinion on whether you or they would benefit from treatment, if symptoms last for more than two weeks.

> One ever-confident man, looking after his wife with dementia, never thought he'd get depressed, but when life got just too 'dark' he finally went to his doctor. The doctor didn't see him as 'weak and useless' as he'd labelled himself. The doctor diagnosed depression. That helped. Having a name for what he was feeling, and the treatment helped, too.

Dysthymia is the name given to mild depression: if untreated its symptoms can become more severe and eventually major, chronic and long-lasting.

Just as dementia is not a personality failing, but rather the result of organic or biochemical changes, so depression often has biochemical origins. Taking medication for depression is the same as taking medication for any other physical problem – asthma, blood pressure and so on. Discuss with your doctor whether an antidepressant may be useful. It must be compatible with other medications, and not make hallucinations and dementia worse in your charge. Be aware also that antidepressants may take a month or so to lift a deep depression.

Deal positively with your feelings
'I' messages

'I' messages are essential for good relationships. When your feelings are hurt, you can use this method to give feedback to anyone in a positive fashion: 'I felt [name the feeling] when you [describe precisely and factually what they were doing].' Practise using them with your charge and anyone else: doctors, helpers, tradespeople. They can't contradict your feelings, and if you describe their behaviour accurately (and they know it) they can't contradict that either.

Sometimes it is appropriate to continue: 'And what I should like to happen is...' You know what you want to happen, and you have let them know without putting them down or attacking them personally. You have not done what so many people do, which is to use 'you' messages such as 'You're a hard-hearted so-and-so' or 'You never take any notice of what I am saying'. Calling the other person names, swearing at them or accusing them of being selfish, opinionated, mean or untidy, can lead to fierce denials, outrage and/or bitterness, instead of solutions.

It is preferable to let them know, using 'I' messages, how what they are doing is affecting you: 'Oh, I wish you'd let me cut up your chicken for you. I get so frustrated when you won't let me because – oh well, you can see the lumps of it on the floor!'

Misunderstandings

Many of our feelings arise because we misunderstand what actually happened, why it happened and what we thought we heard, and we don't clarify it at the time. So, if you say to the person you are with, 'I heard you say [repeat what you think they said], is that right?', you may uncover a different meaning from what you first understood.

Problem-solving

Using 'I' messages is a great introduction to solving problems. The following steps are an extension of the basic idea:
1. Ask the person involved please to listen and help you solve a problem you have.
2. Describe factually what happened – and how this makes you feel.
3. After your input, the other person agrees to cooperate (you hope!) and then you begin 'solving'.
4. Find a pen and paper and sit down together. One of you writes a

list of all the possible solutions you both suggest – even the hilarious ones – with neither of you making any comments.
5. When neither person can think of any more solutions, go through the suggestions one by one together, with a minimum of debate, marking each with a tick or cross.
6. Select one you both agree to try first.
7. Set some guidelines, along with a date and time to meet and evaluate how it's working.
8. Meet on that date, agree to continue along the same or adjusted guidelines, or leave it, select another solution from the list and go through the process again.

Although this process takes time, it is remarkably uncomplicated and successful with helpers, family, health professionals, anyone. It could be a wonderful new life-skill you acquire. But be aware your charge may not be 'together' enough to participate fully.

Sharing your feelings with your charge

Tell your charge about your feelings if this helps. If someone else upsets you, for instance, you may find that telling the person you look after helps you and also helps them feel useful. Sharing in this way also sets them an example of talking about feelings that are upsetting. If you are affected by family or work problems, the person you are looking after may pick up your 'vibes' and be upset. At that point you might embrace them, or hold their hand and say: 'You felt awful when [you heard us quarrelling/ when we were angry with each other/when you heard the bad news about the company].'

Try not to show anger: it is only a by-product of your other stirred-up feelings of impatience, frustration and so on. When you find yourself responding inappropriately, and erupting impatiently with your charge, simply hug them and say you're sorry. They will not remember tomorrow, or even later today.

Accept the frustration, sadness, worry, discouragement, exhaustion or other related feelings that you can identify, and tell them that you are doing your best. Acknowledge your feelings and theirs, and reassure them that you still care for them, and that they are not part of your problems. This can calm them.

Other tips for dealing with feelings
- Say out loud the words for the feelings you can identify. This will give more relief than swearing.
- Keep up to date with your journal. Write out your fears, frustrations and feelings regularly.
- Forgive yourself for not being perfect.
- Find others with whom you can share your experiences.

Sharing experiences
There are many different ways to share your feelings with others to ensure you do not bottle them up:
- Talk about your day's or week's pent-up feelings to a family member, or an understanding neighbour – someone who will listen long and sympathetically.
- Enrol in a carers' education programme offered by your dementia-related organisation. Carers have reported feeling the lifting of heavy burdens and reduction of anxiety and depression as a result.
- Join – or even form – a support group (see Chapter 10: Wider Support and Self-care, 'Support groups'). From such a group you may learn that there is no right way to feel when dealing with dementia. You may see how important it is to recognise how you are feeling, because your feelings affect your reactions – your judgement, your decisions and the care you provide.
- Write thoughts in your journal as memory-prompts and take them to your group.

Sharing feelings, and how you get on top of negative ones, provides you with some relief and can give the other carers valuable tips.

> After all the husbands had been diagnosed with Lewy body dementia, Helen and Donald, Virginia and Drew, Win and Tubby, and Judy and Alan used to meet regularly for drinks and nibbles. They called themselves the Movers and Shakers and had hilarious

times. They didn't talk about their diseases: they talked and laughed about anything and everything else.

'Lewy' made its presence felt increasingly and the absences began – one of the husbands would be in hospital after a fall or another would be in respite care – but the remainder would not think of missing their get-togethers.

Donald died first, after a year in full-time care. Drew died five months later, by which time Alan and Tubby were also being looked after in hospital. Their wives continued to meet, however: the solid support system they had built up over the years made them feel they could face anything.

Everyone needs support in important matters, so seek help in one of the ways suggested above. You'll be setting a great example of being human.

Humour

Laughter is a must. It is said that having two good laughs a day is healthy, with physical benefits such as an all-over body workout and reduction of blood pressure. It certainly makes people feel better.

Most carers feel that if they don't laugh about things, they'll cry, which is another good reason to give laughter a go. Various carers have reported incidents that could have prompted either response, but where they decided to laugh:

Your 80-year-old mother was standing on the bed swatting non-existent flies at 2 am.

◆

Before I went to work, I would sit her at the table and ask her to make me a sandwich to take with me, and to put the cat's breakfast in her dish. I remember, once, when tea break came at work, trying to eat my cat-food sandwich. I often wonder if Fluffy enjoyed her cheese and pickle.

◆

She turned on every element on the stove. I don't know how many hours they glowed so beautifully in the dark.

◆

He said there was no hot water for washing up. He had the cold tap on.

Some people with dementia chuckle and laugh quite easily. Most don't, especially if they have the deadpan face of Parkinsonism. But laughter can be a tonic for the person with dementia as well as their carer.

> Rupert sadly helped Katherine into the car for the trip to her permanent care facility. She was wearing her favourite blue hat for the occasion, but bumped her head slightly as she got in, knocking the hat over her eyes. She looked so ludicrous that Rupert couldn't stop himself. He laughed loudly. 'Oh, Rupert, darling,' Katherine said, turning to him, 'I love it when you laugh!'

◆

> Celia looked after Selwyn in her usual thorough way. She thought he lacked for nothing. But one day after a visiting neighbour departed, having gossiped and chuckled her way through a good half hour, Selwyn said to Celia, 'What a breath of fresh air she is. How good to have all that laughter for a change.' Celia noted his comment and tried to be more light-hearted in future.

Spirituality

Believers and non-believers alike seem to experience spiritual feelings at times. There are said to be few atheists sheltering in bomb craters in wartime; and both the carer and the person they are looking after may find their beliefs shift after a bombshell diagnosis of dementia.

If you are a regular churchgoer, your faith may be shaken.

> My dad's got Alzheimer's. Why him? He doesn't deserve it. I blame God. He caused it. I've stopped going to church, I've stopped reading the Bible, and I've even stopped praying. It doesn't do any good. Nothing seems to do any good.

◆

> Another woman, whose 'wonderful' husband had changed considerably, said, 'I just can't bear to talk about a god any more.'

For some people, however, awareness of a spiritual dimension helps during the dementia journey. One such person said that prayer is their only resource. They prayed quite a bit, and didn't know how they could possibly exist without it.

And from someone with dementia came this clear and thoughtful comment:

> I thank God for trusting me enough to give me such a wonderful opportunity for spiritual growth as I know very well there is no such thing as a bad thing ... it is completely our choice whether to make ourselves miserable or happy by whether we choose to view events as bad or good. For example, if there is a rock in our path, the rock is neither bad nor good. What makes the situation bad or good is whether we stumble over the rock or use it as a stepping stone.

If you have no religious associations you may find yourself upset, lost, even wondering whether having a god would help. As you experience the challenges of dementia, you may be attracted to your local church, synagogue or mosque, and the person you are looking after may benefit from contact with a minister, rabbi, pastor or imam, especially if those people will come to the home. Singing hymns, chanting, joining in prayers out loud, can sometimes overcome your charge's aphasia (loss of power of speech or writing) and make them feel good.

There can, of course, be deep spirituality without organised religion. It can be part of a holistic perspective, as in a traditional Maori approach to life that values maintaining the health of the spirit (wairua), mind (hinengaro), body (tinana) and family (whanau).

If organised religion is not for you, you and/or your charge may find spiritual support by:

- attending retreat centres that have workshops on important issues
- reading about, or taking up meditation, yoga or other spiritual activities
- listening to uplifting music
- studying nature, spiritual art, sacred objects and the like.

Current research about well-being consistently shows that 'spirituality' enhances people's lives, so encourage the person you are caring for to talk about their spiritual feelings. More broadly, reminisce about things in their lives (or your life) which have held great meaning, or about which they (or you) may feel anger, sadness, guilt or gladness. A fresh look at old memories may lead to new understandings and, perhaps, peace.

Where to from here
- Chapter 10: Wider Support and Self-care
- Chapter 13: Communication
- Chapter 14: Intimacy, Love and Sex, especially 'Sex and feelings'
- Chapter 24: Aggression
- Chapter 26: Moving into Full-time Care, especially 'Feelings and reactions'
- Chapter 27: Final Days

Chapter 13

Communication

As we get older some of us have trouble finding the odd word, but we generally understand what is being said, and we don't take an uncomfortably long time to reply. A person with dementia does, however. Hesitations increase and conversation becomes complicated.

Those who have dementia want to be part of things, but they say that having a conversation is like sorting through words lying scattered on the floor to find ones that mean what they are trying to say. And most people around them don't make it easy. They interrupt and won't wait. As one person with dementia noted:

> I wish people would give me time to speak. I search around for the words I want to use and people finish my sentences, guessing what I want to say. I wish they'd just listen – and not make me embarrassed if I lose the thread of what I am saying.

Often people begin avoiding the person who is having difficulties.

Eight ways to be empathetic and helpful

1. Use short, simple sentences.
2. Go on to the next important point only when you know your listener has taken in the previous one.
3. Keep questions to a minimum and ask them one at a time.
4. Be patient while you wait for an answer. With dementia, people take longer to process information. Half a minute can seem like five minutes, but you will usually get a reply which makes some sort of sense.

5. Chat in a relaxed way about memories and prior accomplishments.
6. Be as polite as you would be with any other friend.
7. Laugh often.
8. Listen carefully. Try to listen twice as much as you talk.
   A woman with dementia told her doctor she hardly talked to her husband any more. 'I don't talk because no one listens.'

Is everything in working order?

You would be wise to check that 'personal aids' are in good working order and to arrange regular, general physical check-ups for your charge, and for yourself, too.

Hearing aids

Hearing loss makes communication harder. The person you are caring for may need a hearing aid, or to have the present one upgraded, or wax in their ears cleared out.

> Tim had become quite apathetic only a few months after his dementia diagnosis. Previously quiet, he became even more so, gazing into space while people around him chatted. They gave up trying to shout anything but essentials to him. His wife Greta thought that, mentally, he was slipping back quite quickly.
>
> At his quarterly hearing test, she reported cleaning his hearing aids daily, and replacing the little batteries frequently. However, the audiologist was appalled by the wax in both ears. 'He wouldn't have been able to hear anything!' he said.
>
> Once his ears were cleaned, Tim was a different man.

People happily wear glasses – so why do they object to using hearing aids? They are not perfect, but they make life easier in the long run – for the wearer and for those around them. Perhaps your doctor could persuade the person you look after (or you) to try one.

Other suggestions if the person you are caring for is deaf:

✦ Obtain amplification on your phone; communication can be particularly difficult when the listener has no visual clues from the person talking.

- Use email or a fax machine. It allows time for them to understand messages and respond at their own speed.

However, don't be too optimistic – it may be that what is deteriorating is their ability to understand rather than their hearing, and they may find electronic equipment too difficult to adjust to.

Other aids

- Check their dentures. Badly fitting dentures can make talking difficult and make eating messy and painful.
- Check their prescription for glasses. They may be losing the ability to convert the symbols they see into words and meaning; but they may simply not be able to see properly.
- Have large cards with frequently used names and phone numbers in clear figures near each phone, so they can ring family and friends more easily. Voice amplifiers, pacing boards (which help slow down speech), portable typing devices and alphabet charts (to spell out words that are difficult to say clearly) are available. Ask your therapist or support organisation about them.

Medications and other health problems

Sometimes the medication your charge is taking can affect their ability to communicate. However, deterioration in communication can also signal another health problem. Tell your doctor of any significant or abrupt changes in how your charge communicates.

Speech and language therapy

Courses in speech and language therapy can help some people with dementia. Others refuse that sort of course, be it physiotherapy, exercises, or lectures on their condition. Rather than trying to change their behaviour, you may do better to develop coping strategies.

Managing communication difficulties

Part of caring for a person with dementia means taking them out with other people and keeping their lives as normal as possible. But you may find in general conversation that others often can't be bothered waiting, or think the person with dementia is not able to respond, or become embarrassed by the silence. Maybe they think it's not worth trying and move off, or talk to someone else. All these responses will be wounding for your companion, but you can prevent or manage the situation in several ways.

Relax – and encourage others to relax – if your companion is slow in conversation. Let them speak for themselves. They have a right to express their opinions and it is important that their concerns are aired. Listen to yourself: do you wait to hear what they are saying, or are you uncomfortable with silences?

If someone asks your companion a question, try not to answer for them, even if they take a long time to reply. Wait those extra 15 seconds and, maybe, ask the questioner to wait, too. You could say, in an encouraging voice, 'Take your time. It's not easy, but we'll wait.'

> After George died, their doctor said to his wife, 'I learned a lot from you, Beverley.'
>
> This surprised and pleased her, and she couldn't resist asking, 'What was that, Doctor?'
>
> 'I noticed the way you said nothing and waited for George to answer, when I asked him questions. I learned to wait, too, because he usually told me eventually what I wanted to know – or he'd ask you to reply for him.'

If your companion replies to a question in a garbled way, it might help to paraphrase what you believe they are trying to say. Ask them, 'Is that what you wanted me/us to hear?' Have a signal arranged with them in case they want you to help them out, but definitely don't talk for them unless they ask you.

Don't explain everything to them; it slows down the conversation. It is better to assume they are listening and understanding.

Avoid talking across them to another person as though they were not there, and never say anything you would not want them to hear. In the later stages of their disease it will be impossible to know how much they hear or understand, because their comprehension may vary from minute to minute.

Be aware that whispering or laughing around them may be misinterpreted. However there is no misinterpreting the use of 'we', as often heard in nursing homes: 'We have to go to bed now', 'How about we wear these shoes today?' It is simply degrading.

Making yourself understood
Keep it simple
Radio, television and background noises should ideally be absent, or kept to a minimum. If your companion is hard of hearing, keep on the same eye level, lean towards them and speak clearly. Make sure you look relaxed.

Introduce your topic. Your first few words in a sentence are important, because they give the person with dementia a lead-in to what you are about to say. Use few words and be specific: 'Come and get into the car' is more effective than 'Now it's time to go and see the doctor'. On the other hand, simple and general terms are better than complex vocabulary; say 'the neighbour's car' instead of 'the neighbour's Holden station-wagon'.

You are safest to avoid colloquialisms or idiomatic expressions like 'Jump into the car now.' The hearer is likely to take it literally and might be alarmed that you want them to be so energetic. Likewise it is best not to make jokes or funny comments, or try to be too clever in conversation.

Take it step by step
When doing routine tasks with your charge or organising events or outings, try using one-step-at-a-time instructions to make it easier for them. Use identical words each time, repeating a step several times, if necessary.

> The family of an always imperious mother with developing dementia had arranged a special dinner for her birthday. She was all ready for it, when she suddenly said she didn't feel up to it, and went and lay on her bed, fully dressed.
>
> Soon her son came and stood by her bed. 'You're not feeling too well, Mum,' he said sympathetically. She grunted. 'Let's see how well or bad you are feeling. See if you can put just one foot on the ground.' She frowned, pushed herself up and dropped one leg down until her foot rested on the carpet. 'Good. Now see if you

can put the other foot beside it.' She pushed herself further up to sit and put the other foot down. 'Right. That's good. Now you can sit up properly. How about seeing if you can stand?' He put his arm around her back and she stood up. 'That's great. Now see if you can walk across the room.'

He walked her around the room while he chatted. She was visibly cheering up. He said, 'See, you're able to make it to dinner after all,' and he helped her downstairs to where the family waited.

She really enjoyed the evening.

If even short, simple steps are not understood, try using different key words or showing visually what you want the person to do. Point with your finger. Use your arms and hands to demonstrate. Hold up, and waggle to make them see, the trousers you want them to put on. When dementia is more advanced, pointing, demonstrating or guiding an action may be more helpful than trying to explain verbally.

Forget about being self-conscious; but be aware that your charge may not remember and you may have to do it all again tomorrow. If the person you're talking to still can't understand, give up if it's not very important. Don't get into a fight. Have a good laugh together.

When cooperation is necessary, spend time chatting about the task before you approach it, whether it is showering, exercising, getting ready for bed, or going to the doctor. Make requests in a light-hearted, encouraging way, rather than ordering or demanding.

Slow down to your charge's speed and keep them informed as to what stage they are at. For instance, 'That's you all washed and clean so it's time to dry you. Okay, now come through and get dressed.'

Speak slowly and calmly, and be aware they will notice your non-verbal language if it is the opposite of your words. Use 'I' messages (see Chapter 12: Feelings), and be patient while they take time to understand you.

They may cooperate and manage faster actions if you ask them nicely – and not often.

Right from the start of Trevor's decline, Connie had adopted patience as her motto, but one day they were running extremely late for their lunch date with friends because she'd had to do a complete change of his clothes after one of his 'toilet accidents'.

'Hey, Trev,' she said cheerfully, 'I've got a few things still to do before we leave. Could you hurry up and get yourself into the car? We're running terribly late.'

To her amazement Trevor galloped at almost three times his usual pace down the hall, out the door and got himself into the car – but she decided not to push her luck by trying it too often.

Understanding a person with dementia

You may discover you can make sense of the person's choice of words by:
- finding links between words – a banana can become 'a nice thing you put in your mouth' or 'a yellow cucumber'
- looking for attitudes or emotions behind the words
- using imagination and guesswork!

One woman called anything small with four legs 'little bears' (like her old teddy bear). Don't correct such a description; someone with dementia won't remember. Say, 'Yes, isn't it soft and cuddly?'

Words that come out of your charge's mouth are rarely meaningless. Be aware of their age and background when trying to make sense of their words. Language changes with each generation. The words they are using may be obsolete now.

Ask other family members about possible meanings. Sometimes families talk in codes; if you are an outside carer, you may miss meanings the family would understand. Language from childhood may reappear in the person's vocabulary, and, although you may have known them for decades, they may have had their early years elsewhere.

If they use childish words like 'wee-wee' or 'tinkle', do not treat them as children. If what they say is garbled, apologise with a smile and ask them to say it again. Say, 'It's very tiring getting me to understand. Keep on trying. I want to know.'

Maintain a caring atmosphere and encourage them as you would someone trying to speak a new language. Remember the person is not purposely being difficult to hear or understand.

In a questioning tone, come up with a key word you think you heard your charge say. Try to create a sentence or two from their words. If they nod to show that is what they meant, add another sentence and ask whether that is correct.

As you would wait and help someone in pain or on crutches, recognise what an effort it is for the person trying to talk. Wait and help.

Common irritations
Repetition

Repeating the same question or statement is extremely common. Your charge might tell you about the same incident time and again, or keep asking you 'When's lunch?' Never reprimand them. Keep calm and patient. Just answer the same each time: 'At a quarter past twelve – in half an hour.' This saves you having to think up something new or different to say.

Repetition is their way of letting you know that they have forgotten what you said the first time, or they may not have remembered having asked before. They may be feeling insecure, abandoned, frightened.

Try to identify their possibly troubled feeling and respond: 'You're a bit upset. I'll take care of you. I'll see that you get your meal. It'll be at a quarter past twelve. Don't worry, I'm here.'

Alternatively you can write a reply and put it in a prominent place, for example 'Lunch will be at 12.15 pm.' Gesture towards the note next time they ask.

Sometimes the person may repeat something intentionally:
One carer did say mildly to the person she was looking after, that she had asked the same question about the grandchildren several times, to which the response was, 'Oh, it gives me such comfort to hear myself saying their names over and over.'

Echoing

Your charge echoes back to you what you have said to them or speaks fragments of it. They have apparently heard what you said but are obviously having difficulty in responding. Try being imaginative and suggest responses they might be trying to make.

Disagreement

Argument is counter-productive. At some point people with dementia will no longer be able to reason, will not remember any points you make, and will probably only get cross. Agree instead.

What your charge says is their reality. If they say 'I'm going to New York next week,' say something like: 'Okay, can I see about the bookings for you?' or 'How nice. I wonder who you'll meet there that I know.'

If they become annoyed despite all your efforts, try the following:
- Admit that you are both getting nowhere.
- Accept their feelings if they become abusive and aggressive verbally (see Chapter 24: Aggression).
- Apologise.
- Drop the subject.
- Use distraction; offer a snack.

Avoid becoming angry and aggressive yourself. Move away if necessary and come together another time.

Strokes and communication

If your charge has had a bad stroke, they will probably be paralysed on one side of their body and their dementia may have increased. Alternatively, their remaining mental powers may be unimpaired but they may be unable to speak because of paralysis or other problems. Signals become all-important.

> Lydia had a bad stroke and spent two months deeply unconscious in hospital until, one day, her brother saw her eyes open.
>
> She made no response at all to his excited talk so he tried another strategy. 'Lydia, it's Ron here. I'm so glad to see your eyes open, but I'm sad you can't talk. How about giving me a signal? If you can hear what I'm saying, give me a signal and shut your eyes and keep them shut for a few seconds.'
>
> To his delight, Lydia's eyes shut and stayed closed. 'Lydia, that's absolutely fabulous! You can open them again now.'
>
> Lydia's eyes opened again, and that was the beginning of her 'getting better'. But she came out of hospital with 'vascular

dementia', and communicated as well as she could in the future with nods and shakes of the head, smiles and down-turned mouth.

Make contact with your local stroke organisation, and experiment with signals using hands, fingers, eyebrows, eyes, noses, grunts and whistles, and so on. Your charge's brain may still be active, and there could be exciting results.

Diminishing verbal abilities

In dementia, verbal communication abilities deteriorate in roughly the following order:
1. They are unable to remember names, thoughts or memories.
2. They use the wrong word, mispronounce or repeat words, or invent words.
3. They have difficulty organising thoughts, are distracted.
4. They lose speed in their reasoning ability for taking part in friendly debate.
5. They fall back on language that is very direct, accusatory or indecent.
6. They use more non-verbal gestures, become withdrawn and speak very little.
7. They are very difficult to understand because of distorted speech. Often they don't take in enough breath to complete what they were saying, or they know what they want to say but it doesn't come out right.
8. They appear bored or not interested because of little variation in the pitch of their voice and a 'mask-like' facial expression. Let people know this is not so.
9. They find it increasingly difficult to describe problems they want to tell you about.

Bruce, spending two weeks in respite care, was sitting in the day room when Alison arrived after lunch. He saw her and waved urgently.

When she took his hand it was icy cold. In the middle of winter he had on only a long-sleeved shirt and tracksuit pants – and no socks, just slip-on leather moccasins.

'You're so cold, darling,' she exclaimed. 'You need more clothes on. Why didn't you ask for more clothes when you were being dressed?' Alison realised she shouldn't have asked: Bruce now couldn't make those requests for himself.

She walked with him through to his room, turned the heater on to high and wrapped him up in lots of warm clothes while he sat thawing out, vacant and vulnerable in his armchair.

Communicating with a hospital resident

Approach the person with dementia from the front, so as not to startle them. Give them a wave and a smile and come closer slowly, to give them time to know that you're coming to see them (this also lets you gauge their mood).

Say who you are; show you're pleased to see them: hugs, kisses and squeezes can establish warmth and friendship. They like to feel you still want to chat to them, so have a few items of gossip ready, and make sure you stay more than a minute or two. Don't seem to be in a hurry; relax if possible.

Have an opening 'ritual' prepared; maybe a gift of a piece of fruit (though sometimes the home will not want you to feed them just before a meal) or a flower. This gives you something else to talk about, as you put it in a vase.

Get to know the person's 'at rest' facial expression, so that you can detect changes which indicate their mood. If you receive a hostile reception and it persists, retreat and try again later. Half an hour can produce quite a different response.

If you visit during an organised activity which they are watching or are involved in, don't interrupt, just wait unobtrusively.

Hilda saw her old friend, Jim, sitting in a large circle of fellow patients when she went to visit him. She found a chair away from the group out of his sight, and sat watching.

The two teams playing skittles were as competitive as any other teams you would find. They cheered, laughed, teased and sang team songs to lift their side's morale.

Hilda realised how many friends Jim had, especially one woman who fussed around him. Indeed, when Hilda went up to him at the end of the game, this woman said, 'Oh, you're not coming to take my Jim away from me, are you? He's my special fella!'

When the person no longer speaks
They can still communicate

Look for non-verbal communication. Guess and suggest what their unspoken messages might be. If they begin to wander, it may be an attempt to let people know that they need something, so make sure they are getting enough food, drink and rest. General restlessness and agitation may be caused by toothache, pain, indigestion, toilet needs, thirst or sheer boredom. Listening skills may help you identify the cause.

Sometimes you can agree to signals: a squeeze of the hand can mean 'I like things this way', or a wave of the hand can mean 'No. Stop.'

Be aware of your own stance, facial expression, tension and so on. They will be sensitive to your tone of voice and body language.

You may still get their attention

Look directly at the person you are visiting. Make sure you have their attention. If you can't get it, wait a few minutes and try again. Move slowly and gently. Touch an arm or a hand. Say their name several times. Keep at eye level with them, especially if they are very disabled or deaf. Usually this means sitting down, leaning towards them and looking relaxed.

> Loretta, a keen gardener in her time, was bedridden in hospital and really going downhill. Her sister-in-law, Ngaire, visited and brought a large bunch of highly perfumed flowers.
>
> Loretta, propped up in bed, went on staring into space, but Ngaire spoke her name softly several times, and moved the flowers up and down and from side to side in front of her until the scent and colours tweaked Loretta's senses. Her eyes began to move and her nose to twitch. She smiled.
>
> Ngaire moved the flowers until Loretta's eyes focused first on them, then on Ngaire, at which point Ngaire laid the flowers on the

bed. There was a sort of recognition from Loretta, another smile, and a mutual squeeze as their hands joined. Loretta did not speak as her visitor chatted away, but Ngaire felt she had communicated with her and her visit had been a poignant success.

Keep talking

Keep on talking to them. Don't overload them, but realise that their inability to talk doesn't mean they don't want to hear your voice. If they are profoundly deaf you may feel the need to talk loudly, which can tire you – but be aware that the 'murmur' as your voice comes through can be comforting.

Tell them their family news and your own, and other local chat. Use facial expressions and hand gestures to clarify what you are saying.

Use physical touch

Communicate with lots of physical touch, if appropriate (some people dislike physical contact), to convey your friendship and empathy.

- ✦ Sit close and hold their hand.
- ✦ Give hugs, lay a supportive hand on their arm when walking, put your arm around a shoulder, brush their hair, stroke their cheek.
- ✦ Squeeze their hand gently, perhaps with a gentle massage. This is valuable unspoken communication.

Activities are a way to 'talk'

Communicate with gentle activities: sing a favourite song or hymn, quote a familiar saying, or accompany them on a walk around the garden or street. You are showing that you accept them.

> When her mother stopped talking, one daughter found it difficult and stressful carrying on a one-sided conversation. Then she began bringing flowers from her mother's garden to the hospital. Chatting about the flowers as she arranged them made the time pass much more easily. Later her mother loved it when the daughter began quietly manicuring her hands. It was comfortable, tactile communication.

Laughter helps
Laugh often. Laughter helps reduce strain for everyone. Use humour, cajoling, or gentle teasing at difficult moments.

> Trevor refused to take food or drink. Connie tended him gently, speaking to him quietly as he sat in his wheelchair, moistening his dry lips and sitting beside him, not knowing what else she could do for him. Bertha, a nursing sister, came up to ask how they were getting on. Hearing Connie's response, she chuckled, leaned in and said, 'Oh, that's not good enough, Trevor!'
>
> Very deaf, he gave no indication that he had heard.
>
> 'Hey, Trevor man,' Bertha said in a very loud voice, leaning further. She laughed loudly and ruffled his bearded cheek with her fingers. 'Trevor, my love, I've got your drink here – just what you're waiting for.'
>
> Trevor looked around, beamed and pursed his lips to take the drinking beaker she offered.
>
> Connie had been too shy to talk and laugh loudly, she realised, because there were other people around.

When you have important information
You are trying to prevent 'loss of self' in the person with dementia, so, although they really can't talk, make sure:
- they are told necessary information
- they understand important decisions
- you go over it with them in printed form if possible.

If they get confused, say, 'This is hard for you to take in. I'll repeat that', and say the same words simply and clearly.

Watch their non-verbal communication for signs of agreement, disagreement or discomfort. If they are physically uncomfortable, this may take their mind off what you are talking about.

Ask the person with dementia fairly often whether they understand. Take their nods or shakes of the head as appropriate 'Yes' or 'No' answers.

Be patient when you're not sure whether they understand; and if you decide finally that they can't follow your verbal attempts, try a physical movement instead to illustrate what you want to get across.

Leave it, if it's not absolutely important. This is when an enduring power of attorney may prove useful.

Practice and patience

Communication is very important, but it is very difficult to put these skills, involving so much patience, into practice. We can only try.

> 'I failed in this area many times, in spite of trying very hard,' said one carer, 'and I had to deal with lots of guilt from feeling impatient and bossy.'

Where to from here

- Chapter 12: Feelings, especially '"I" messages'
- Chapter 14: Intimacy, Love and Sex
- Chapter 26: Moving into Full-time Care, especially 'When they don't speak'

Chapter 14

Intimacy, Love and Sex

Catering for intimacy and love

We all need moments of intimacy and to feel liked and accepted. Carers and their charges who still live in a marriage have this – in theory, at least – with daily confirmation of their continuing worth and of being loved.

For couples who have grown apart or who no longer sleep together because of the disruptions of dementia, intimacy and affection are less easily achieved but can be close at hand. For people with dementia who live on their own, visitors provide the only close human contact that can fulfil these needs.

Pets and affection

Stroking a cat, dog, or even a rabbit, may help the person you are looking after to meet some of their needs for affection, warmth and touch. Consider having a pet – even a neighbour's dog – for your charge to walk, groom, feed and watch, as well as cuddle or stroke. You would, of course, have to ensure good care, with suitable food, housing, warmth, a clean environment and protection from possible rough handling.

Catering for sexual needs

The wide variety of attitudes towards sex in the community makes it inappropriate to offer carers definite advice about catering for their charges' sexual needs – or their own. The general guidelines used throughout this book apply as well to sexual needs: be as patient as possible, accept respectfully the person behind their mask of dementia, and balance their needs fairly against your own.

Most people manage their sex lives doing what (they think) comes naturally. But their interpretation of 'natural' is moulded – enhanced, constrained, inhibited – by their own earlier experiences, and by family attitudes and habits, rather than by nature or the Kama Sutra. Lecturers and writers on dementia usually give little help, often skimming over the sexual aspects of the condition. Perhaps the subject embarrasses them, or perhaps they assume the sexual desires of older people disappear along with their hair, muscles and memory. You and the person you are looking after are individuals, and respond best when you both have your needs met. Reading about others' experiences in this chapter may help you sort out your own expectations and solutions.

When you and your charge are partners

If the person you are looking after is your sexual partner, you may find sex doesn't change after a dementia diagnosis.

> A wife, whose husband's dementia had come on fairly quickly, was surprised that it hadn't changed their sex life at all. 'Nothing has changed in that department,' she said.

But that is not everybody's experience. With dementia intruding, and perhaps also depression or medication side-effects, new or greater challenges may surface. These could involve differences with desire, physical difficulties, inability to show sensitivity or emotion, failure to recognise a partner or remember shared experience, the attractions of a third party, difficult behaviour in public, or discussion of sex and feelings. Any of these might be demanding or distressing, but occasionally there is a funny side.

> Connie was granted helpers to look after Trevor three mornings a week. After the middle-aged, competent, friendly and very attractive brunette had visited a few times, Connie thought she was great, but Trevor said, 'She's not suitable. We'll have to send her back.'
> 'Why, Trev? She seems very good, and nice with it.'
> 'That's it, Con. She's too attractive!'

Intimacy, Love and Sex   157

Different levels of desire

Different levels of desire can bring challenges and changes. Previously accepted patterns of lovemaking may change if the person with dementia loses their inhibitions and demands gratification, for instance. For one couple, this was positive.

> Katya had dementia and was continually frustrated because she could hardly get her words out, and needed a lot of help to get through her day; but her husband was very understanding and supportive. His attentions seemed to stimulate her sexual desires, which pleased him greatly.

Not all partners are able to respond like this, though. Sometimes the sexual urge disappears when the role of carer starts to dominate, or if other health issues emerge.

> Dorothy and Ed, her husband of 33 years, stoically continued their lives much as before her Alzheimer's diagnosis. That included their love life, although Ed had diabetes which affected his potency. But well into Dorothy's illness she quite suddenly became sexually very demanding. Every night she clung and pleaded. Ed did what he could to satisfy her, but it all became too much for him and he had to seek help from their doctor.

The wife in another couple found that she had lost all desire once she became her husband's main carer. Although she was still very fond of him and was sure he still loved her, she was so busy managing everything that she had no time or energy left over when he made sexual advances. 'It's just not the same as before. I'm too busy thinking about how to manage things.'

Memory loss

Memory loss may mean some people with dementia feel they never get enough sex, just as some repeatedly ask when dinner will be, even just after eating.

> 'Carlo's sex drive seems to be increasing at the same rate that his memory is decreasing,' complained his wife. 'He gets quite aggressive if I turn him down, and I'm getting worn out. I tried to

> get him to understand my feelings, and got him to agree to only
> every two or three days. But he'd forgotten this by the next day and
> began pestering me again.'

One way to deal with this could be to have a signed contract (see Chapter 6: Becoming a Carer, 'Making a contract'). The wording might be interesting!

Memory loss can also result in your partner forgetting an arrangement you've made together. If a planned-for sexual event does not happen, nobody may be the worse for it.

> Connie tried to keep Trevor happy by offering sex every month or
> so, after he developed dementia. He would respond with interest,
> although his deadpan face didn't show any emotion, so she would
> give him half a Viagra tablet and sit with him watching television
> until the time was ripe. But more than once he forgot what they
> had been planning and said, 'Oh, I don't think so. Not now!' Connie
> didn't actually mind at all.

Women and men

Men often retain their interest in intercourse far longer than women. Erections, with or without dementia, go on and on.

> Some days Greta would be woken early by Tim's hand shaking her
> shoulder. He would be standing by her bed with a 'morning glory': it
> was obvious what he was hoping.
>
> Trying to conceal her lack of interest, she would wriggle over
> and open the bedclothes and Tim would drop in beside her, stone
> cold, hardly able to move, but longing for some sort of sexual relief.
>
> It was not as it used to be, and often nothing much eventuated,
> as Greta tried to avoid being touched by his icy fingers while she
> stroked his erect penis, but they both felt more positives than
> negatives from the encounter – he, that he had been accepted; she,
> feeling satisfaction for having made the effort.

Desire is not always linked to gender, however, and sometimes women can have more interest in sex than their partners do. Also, sex is no longer a priority for some men with dementia:

Sean had always seemed 'full of sex', but it waned as his Huntington's disease took over. He moved into another bedroom when he began 'thrashing and bicycling around'.

◆

For Ben, interest in sex also drifted away as his dementia increased, but he still seemed to want to show his love in other ways. Sophie, his wife, found she adapted quite well.

◆

Ralph was uncoordinated and often incontinent. He hallucinated regularly and often did not know who his wife, Josie, was, but she regularly hugged Ralph, saying she loved him. At other times, Ralph would suddenly look at Josie and spread his own arms wide. She would walk into them and he would hug her unsteadily and tell her, 'I love you.' This made her feel that her marriage was still there and that all her exhaustion and caring were worthwhile.

Sex and feelings
Your charge's feelings

The person you are looking after may long for affection and closeness, but find this difficult to achieve when their condition restricts physical actions or rigidity prevents sensual movement. They may also feel they have become unattractive; they may fear rejection, lack self-esteem, or be confused about how to express their sexual needs.

They may become jealous about an interest they imagine you show in another, or be suspicious when you come too close, not recognising you. Accept their fears. Reassure them. Remain warm and available. Try to keep constant communication going. Such responses indicate an ideal partner and an ideal carer, but your needs, wants and feelings may affect your ability to act in this way. This complicates life for you.

Your feelings

As both a partner and a carer, you may feel any of a wide range of emotions about sex with the person you are looking after. You may even have conflicting emotions. Rather than immediately dismiss your feelings, recognise them. Then you can more clearly work out what to do.

For instance, if you feel guilt, a need to please, concern about doing what is proper and so on, you might note this in your journal – without judgement – before you decide what action to take. If such feelings arise from your upbringing, think about whether they need to influence what you do in your current relationship.

You may feel frustrated or depressed if you have continuing and unfulfilled sexual needs, leading to such responses as:

- initiating sex when you feel like it ('Blow it. I'll make the first move for a change!')
- hoping that a prescription such as Viagra might help
- resigning yourself to just forgetting about sex.

Otherwise, your spouse's reduced interest in sex may leave you feeling grateful that those demands have gone.

Some partners who are also carers can find their charge's approaches unpleasant. If sex is far from comfortable for you, you have a right to say no.

> After five years of her husband's Parkinson's there was one aspect of his deterioration Brenda could not cope with – the increasingly expressionless, rough, insensitive approaches he made to her sexually. She knew Adrian loved her. She knew his dementia had robbed him of the sensitivity and sensuality they had long enjoyed, so she tried to let her brain provide the fantasy which would make his 'lovemaking' acceptable.
>
> Eventually, however, Brenda felt so violated that she had to tell Adrian, 'No more.' She said to her confidante, 'It seemed I could've just been a rubber doll as far as he was concerned.'

If your partner's dementia puts you off, you are not a terrible person, nor are you the first. You may – even unexpectedly – find a way through:

> One husband cared lovingly for his wife for months. She developed dementia fairly rapidly, and he found it was hugely demanding coping with her ups and downs. When she was upset he found she responded best if he just patiently held her and stroked her.
>
> After she eventually became incontinent he was unable to face intercourse with her any more. He hated hurting her feelings

when she sometimes suggested plaintively that they go to bed together, but could not summon up any desire. He had to admit it: she smelt. But one morning, as he was drying her after her shower, she had a period of intense agitation and, to his surprise, as he held and stroked her to calm her down, he found himself aroused. He realised, of course, that she was freshly clean and desirable as of old. They made the most of that occasion, and he began looking forward to similar mornings when they could start their old love-making again.

Talking about sex
Talking to your partner

Acknowledging your feelings to yourself is one step. Can you take another step and talk to your partner about a sexual difficulty you have? Here are a few ideas for opening up a conversation with them:

- ✦ This rotten disease makes sex difficult, doesn't it?
- ✦ I never thought we'd have difficulties with our love life till we were in our nineties!
- ✦ I know sex isn't easy for you. Shall we try Viagra?
- ✦ Would you like to make love? It's hard for me to know, these days.
- ✦ I know it's not easy to make love now, but I do so miss it. Could we try?

See 'Intimacy without intercourse' below, for other possibilities that you and your partner could discuss.

Talking with others

There comes a point when the person in your care cannot discuss these things with you – or you may have good reasons not to confide in them. Yet your experiences may feel too painful or too damaging to keep to yourself, as Brenda did in the story above.

Who can you turn to? Sex is considered such a 'private' matter, it may not have occurred to you to talk to anyone else. In fact you won't be the only one: others can have similar problems and find it just as hard to mention them.

If you raise the subject – with your support group, for instance – you may not only feel better for it but also help others with their predicament, or at least show them that they are not alone.

The person you are caring for may also need others to confide in, so try to find someone for them. You may even find that helping them in this way will benefit you too.

A doctor or a counsellor?

Your doctor may (or may not) seem an obvious person to confide in. In fact it is essential to talk to them if you are considering Viagra or similar medications. These should be avoided by people with cardiovascular disease, or who use nitrolingual sprays or other nitrates. Your doctor will know about any possible clashes with an existing condition or other current medication.

If you make a special appointment with your doctor to discuss concerns about sex with your partner with dementia, your doctor may surprise you by being unhelpful and invoking 'patient privacy'. But, as carer, you may need special information and be entitled to it. (See Chapter 7: Dealing with Health Professionals.)

The doctor may prefer you to consult a counsellor, and may be able to suggest one. It is important you feel comfortable with any counsellor and confident in their abilities. Certainly the woman in the following story might have benefited from talking with a skilled professional of this kind:

> Warwick and Sharon began a very happy union in late middle-age, with a love life which enthralled them both. After three years, however, Warwick showed signs of dementia and began making sexual moves at inappropriate times, touching Sharon's breasts in company, for example, but impersonally and without his old warmth. In fact he became obsessively sexual in an unfeeling way. Sharon was upset and wondered whether it was a part of his personality that she hadn't known.

In the case above, the person with dementia went rapidly downhill and into full-time care. This brought a different heartache that a counsellor or support group may have been able to help with.

Other options for physical intimacy

For a couple who wish to be physically intimate, sufficient pleasure may come from simply lying sideways facing each other, kissing and caressing. If this eventually develops into foreplay, intercourse is often easier with the carer on top; but if the other insists on that position, it becomes physical exercise. Lots of wriggling and grunts and puffs result, and laughter does not go amiss.

Intimacy without intercourse

If mutual stimulation or the actual 'congress' is uncomfortable and difficult, other actions may be welcome, preferable and effective.

Looking at the list of intimate acts below, think how you would rank their order of importance to you. If you can, discuss this with your partner, too, and find out which they think are most or least important:

- hugs
- kisses
- arms around waist
- arms around shoulders
- touching when passing
- lying together embracing
- lying together side by side, not embracing
- stroking generally
- spoken declarations of love and/or fondness
- holding hands
- fondling face and hair
- thanks
- penetration
- fondling genitals or breasts
- ejaculation
- stroking erotic zones.

With this exercise, you may discover that for you and/or your partner, intercourse is not the be all and end all.

> Louis and Moira were in their early sixties when he developed
> dementia. Moira says that Louis just ceased being interested in sex

and they hadn't had intercourse since the end of that year. But they still have lots of cuddles and she will jump on him in bed and tell him she's going to 'ravish' him. He loves it!

Be inventive

If you are the healthy partner and you wish to maintain a sex life, you may need to be more active, in ways out of character with your former role in the relationship. This is a time to lose inhibitions, be inventive and look after your own needs too. Some amazing books that you may not have considered reading before, such as David Schnarch's *Passionate Marriage*, can help.

You may also find that self-pleasuring, with or without the knowledge or involvement of your partner, releases some frustrations. In one old educational film, focusing on men's sexual difficulties, a pithy saying was: 'If your wife's not at your right hand, let your right hand be your wife!' Masturbation is also an option for your person with dementia, if they want sex when you don't.

Some carers, for whom intercourse remains vital and whose partners can no longer oblige, will choose another sexual partner. Other carers, who yearn for emotional intimacy, will find it elsewhere:

> I was feeling rather desperate without the old intimacy and friendship that I had with him, so I've had to make do in other directions. Actually, I look now to friends and my family for closeness and I find I get by okay. No sex, of course, but we've become much closer as a family.

If your charge is not your partner

Where there is no sexual relationship, some of the complex feelings discussed above do not arise. However, you may be aware of the sexual needs of the person you are looking after. They may want to talk about and act on their urges, or they may have difficulty talking about and dealing with them.

Think about how you can most effectively give general affection and warmth as well as how to deal with your charge's most intimate needs.

You may, or may not, feel that the carer in the following story did 'the right thing'.

> Gwen had known Horace when they were both working for the same company. Now, many years later, his wife had died and he was left on his own with Parkinson's and increasing dementia. He needed a carer. Gwen was between jobs, had always thought what a fine man he was, and let the extended family know that she was available to look after him. They accepted.
>
> Horace had changed considerably. She found his weakness and dementia appalling, but his sweet nature was still there and she settled in, establishing a routine. He didn't take kindly to being told what to do: he could get furious and aggressive if Gwen tried too hard to get his cooperation, and he sometimes chased her around the house despite his shaky condition. Yet he forgot his anger quickly and she learned to avoid agitating him.
>
> She also became aware of his loneliness – how he missed his beloved Sandra – and she ached to comfort him. One night, after changing him into his pyjamas and brushing his teeth, she slipped into his bed beside him and held him in her arms. He wept, then relaxed and went to sleep. Gwen was going to be careful, but he made no sexual moves – he was actually impotent – and she continued to do this fairly regularly. For her, it became a natural part of caring.

In a hospital setting
Intimacy with your partner

When your long-term partner goes into full-time care, you may miss having them in your bed, and wish to continue your physical intimacy. Usually the staff will cooperate, and you may be able to stay one night a week.

This can become a private time for mutual sexual gratification; or simply for having a bath or shower together. Perhaps you could finish with a massage (feet or hands), applying lotions and/or gently brushing their hair. Maybe what you want is just to sit close enough to touch and hold hands for longer than usual.

Other residents

You may be able to apply your limited experience with dementia to other residents, relate comfortably with them and share your friendship. Don't hesitate to confer with staff, however, if you see something worrying, such as a patient's loss of inhibitions, or an outsider's inappropriate approaches.

The staff may already be dealing with this. Also, they face a wide range of complex challenges every day and usually have good strategies to resolve them. At some facilities, staff and management have worked through these very carefully.

> Stephan and Vanya were in the same residential home and both had dementia. They became very friendly, but when their behaviour became openly sexual in front of the other residents the manager spoke to them and asked them to keep it private and in their bedrooms.
>
> The manager then called a meeting of the staff to see what they thought about the arrangement, and they had a useful discussion about attitudes to sex in the residential home. They agreed that if the adults were both consenting and happy, there should not be an issue, and they included same-sex couples in this understanding. 'Stephan and Vanya are two adults who are free to choose who they socialise with during the daily activities of the home,' they reasoned, 'so they should also be free to choose who they have sex with – but just not in the open!'

Where to from here
✦ Chapter 9: Managing Difficult Behaviour
✦ Chapter 10: Wider Support and Self-care
✦ Chapter 12: Feelings
✦ Chapter 13: Communication
✦ Chapter 26: Moving into Full-time Care

Part Four

Making Life Easier

Chapter 15

Maintaining Health

Medical treatments for cognitive decline

The dementia that is caused by organic brain disease has no cure, but medications may be available to reduce some of the symptoms.

If your doctor seems unhelpful, ask to be referred to the older people's health service at your local hospital or to a memory clinic, if one is available. If the problems are behavioural, ask to be referred to mental health services.

Another option is to approach your local Alzheimer's organisation. They provide help and support for carers, clients and families.

Anticholinesterases

In Alzheimer's disease and Lewy body dementia, anticholinesterases (also known as cholinesterase inhibitors or acetylcholinesterase inhibitors – AChEIs) are the best drugs so far discovered to help with slowing down cognitive deterioration. They do not help everybody with these dementias, and individual drugs in this group may be more or less helpful for individual people.

These drugs are prescribed as Aricept or Donezil (donepezil), Exelon (rivastigmine) and Reminyl (galantamine). They affect the enzyme that clears away a neurotransmitter, acetylcholine. As well as slowing down the loss of cognitive abilities for a period, they can reduce apathy, anxiety and psychosis.

They are expensive and not necessarily covered by government health funding, but a disability allowance may cover some medication costs.

In vascular dementia

Some studies have looked at whether AChEIs can help with vascular dementia, and this research is continuing. However, people with this kind of dementia have other ways to slow its progress: by dealing with underlying conditions – such as high blood pressure and other risk factors for stroke – either through medication or through lifestyle changes.

Cautionary notes
Some common medications may be unsuitable

At first glance antipsychotic drugs, also known as major tranquillisers or neuroleptics, may seem good for controlling the aggression, agitation and hallucinations often found in dementia, and they have been used extensively in some nursing homes. Although they can sometimes be useful as a last resort, in small doses and with close monitoring, their use is not usually advisable: they can increase the risk of stroke or heart attack and can also worsen dementia symptoms. In Lewy body dementia, especially, they can cause very unpleasant, even dangerous, reactions: worsening cognition, heavy sleepiness, increased physical impairment, fever, muscle rigidity and possible kidney failure. Their use should be avoided for people with this dementia. (See Chapter 25: Choosing Full-time Care, 'Use of restraints'.)

Sedatives and minor tranquillisers (different from antidepressants) should likewise be used only as a last resort. They may increase confusion, but can be useful if behaviour becomes very difficult. They may be needed for only a short time, for instance in cases of delirium.

Mobility-enhancing Parkinson's drugs containing levodopa (also known as L-dopa and marketed as Madopar or Sinemet) can also produce unfortunate side-effects: while easing the stiffness of LBD, they can increase the frequency of hallucinations.

> A specialist had diagnosed Norman with Parkinson's disease and had privately advised his doctor that dementia was present too, though Norman and his wife Philippa were not told. The levodopa Norman was given appeared to help his movements a little, but he had hallucinations fairly often, his reading, writing and mental skills continued to diminish, and he found chairing meetings very difficult.

A year later another specialist mentioned Alzheimer's, and later still Norman was told he had Lewy body dementia. Since levodopa can induce hallucinations, and since two distinguishing symptoms of LBD are hallucinations and Parkinsonism, Philippa wondered whether her husband should ever have been on the drug.

Ropinirole and other fairly new drugs known as agonists can have side-effects that result in pathological gambling and other socially disastrous behaviours (known as impulse control disorders) in perhaps 20 per cent of those taking them.

Medical breakthroughs and natural wonders

Don't get excited when you read about 'breakthroughs' in research connected with dementia. For instance, research into stem cell therapy indicates that injured brain cells may be replaceable in the future – but that is far away. Likewise, be cautious about treatments described as 'natural wonders'. These may not have undergone rigorous research and clinical trials, especially in connection with the form of dementia, other health conditions, or the existing medication regimen that your charge has.

Some scientists have speculated that large doses of antioxidants, such as vitamins C and E or selenium, may reduce cell damage associated with memory loss. Vitamin E, however, should be used with caution, and only on the advice of your doctor, because it can thin the blood. Using it at the same time as other anticoagulants (such as aspirin) can be dangerous.

Incompatibilities and side-effects

Incompatibilities between different medications, including over-the-counter products, can also be dangerous. The elderly and people with dementia are especially vulnerable to these incompatibilities and their side-effects. Ask your doctor or pharmacist to check that proposed and existing medications – taken for any health conditions – won't interact adversely with each other.

If you are taking five drugs together (say pills, liquids, eye drops, patches and over-the-counter medication), the risk of a clash is 50 per cent. If you are taking eight or more, it is very likely that at least one of them is being given to treat the side-effects of another. Whenever new remedies are prescribed you have to be ready for new reactions, which can seem like a completely new disease.

Over-medication

Your doctor might be tempted to prescribe something to treat or tone down a fresh side-effect, but you should always question the necessity for more prescriptions. Sometimes not treating a symptom may be safer than trying to fix it with another medication.

The process of administering many different medicines, especially at the same time and for the same disease, is known as polypharmacy. This may mask other warning signs or result in further symptoms, ranging from sleepiness or nausea to dyskinesia (involuntary movements), problems you will need to consult your physician about if they start. This can become a complicated roundabout.

Over-medication can be a real problem for people with dementia, and for the elderly. So, ask about pros and cons if your doctor suggests more medication. Remember, however, that an illogical objection to medication can be dangerous, too.

When a medication is proposed

When a new medication is proposed, take time with your doctor to understand all aspects of the medication, including any side-effects. The following list may be useful. You may like to copy it, leaving room to note the answers, so you can keep the information in your medical folder and refer to it again in the future.

- ✦ What are the potential benefits of this drug?
- ✦ What proportion of people taking it will benefit?
- ✦ When can we expect to see a result?
- ✦ How will we assess the benefits?
- ✦ Where does the proposed dosage level stand in the usual range?
- ✦ How long is it usual to take this drug?
- ✦ How could it interact with anything else being taken (over-the-counter or prescription products)?

- What side-effects can occur?
- How likely are individual side-effects to occur, and for how long?
- What are the other treatment options (pharmaceutical or other) for this problem?
- In which circumstances should we consider other treatments?

Reviewing medications

Every three months ask your doctor for a review of all medications your charge is taking (50 per cent of patients can come off some of their medications after that time), or when common sense suggests it.

> Randall had had Parkinson's and dementia for a long time and finally had to go into a hospital. His family visited regularly. They and he were universally popular, and he settled in well. When he developed pneumonia two years later the family was warned that the end was near, but he 'turned the corner' three days later and survived, though he was much weaker. The family conferred with the doctors: Randall had no quality of life; was it sensible to continue all the drugs he was taking, for all the conditions he was said to have? Everyone decided 'No' and they were stopped. Randall lived for another two years without them.

Your charge's behaviour and their mini mental status examination (MMSE) results, which are assessed at regular meetings with your specialist, will enable you to rate the effectiveness of the AChEI being used (see 'Anticholinesterases' above).

> Sol, on drugs for diabetes, heart problems and depression, was later diagnosed with Alzheimer's, and had Aricept (donepezil) prescribed. He hated having another drug on top of his usual ones and, after a few months, agitated to stop it. His wife thought this could do little harm and took them out of his pill-popping; but, within a few days, she thought she could detect deterioration. Within 10 days she was sure, so told Sol he had to start again. He had noticed his deterioration himself and agreed without demur.

Note that if an AChEI is discontinued for more than a few days and then resumed, your charge needs to start on a reduced dose and work up again.

When a medication is prescribed

If your charge doesn't ask questions, make sure you understand about any new medications prescribed. Ask for clarification if the doctor uses words or phrases you don't understand. Before you leave the pharmacy counter, always make sure you know:

- the names of the medicine (generic and brand)
- how and when to take or use it – for example, before or after food
- how much to take or use
- how long to continue taking or using it
- how to tell if the medicine is working
- if you need to take any special precautions while taking it – avoiding particular foods or drinks, other medicines (over-the-counter or prescribed), or exposure to sunlight
- what to do if particular side-effects or unseen changes occur
- what to do if you miss a dose, or take an extra one
- what could happen if you suddenly stop taking the medicine
- how and where to store the medicine – such as in the refrigerator
- how often and where you can obtain repeats.

Instructions for individual medications can differ considerably. For instance, levodopa (Sinemet or Madopar) can be taken with or without food, while donepezil (Aricept or Donezil) is usually taken once a day at night-time, well after the evening meal. Some drugs can cause nausea if taken on an empty stomach – and some foods can affect medications; for example, certain high-protein foods can affect Parkinson's medications.

Managing medications
Guidelines for taking medication

Every year many people's illnesses get worse, or they end up in hospital, because they did not take their medications properly. Make sure your charge takes all prescribed medications at the set times each day, so that:

- they are less likely to be forgotten
- they maintain steady levels in the bloodstream, which controls symptoms best
- side-effects are less likely.

General advice about what to do if a dose is missed is to take it, providing it is remembered within the hour; otherwise, to skip it and take it at the next scheduled time. Because medications and the people taking them are all different, however, it is best to check with your doctor.

When the person with dementia enters care, managing their medication regimen becomes more complex. Often medications are administered when the staff do their rounds with the medicine trolley, rather than at the set times the person with dementia has been used to. This may be one of the frustrations to be addressed when adjusting to institutional life.

Safekeeping and dispensing

Keep medicines out of children's reach and out of your charge's reach, should their dementia be sufficiently advanced. They must not use other people's medications, or let others use theirs.

Dispose of any medications past their use-by date (your pharmacist can do this for you). But never throw away the labelled container your current medication came in, as you may need it to get a refill or to give proof for reissue.

If the person you are looking after forgets to take medicines, buy a medication holder with a timer that beeps at pre-set times, or a wristwatch alarm. A pharmacy-prepared blister pack or a labelled medicine tray/pill dispenser with compartments are other possible solutions. These can also set you up for the week, avoiding having to fiddle around with different pills out of different containers several times a day. Check the first blister pack to ensure it has been filled correctly.

Prepared packs make dosages and times clear, and with them your charge may be able to take their pills and potions themselves, as long as they can still tell the time and understand the calendar. If they do not know what day of the week it is, you will have to take responsibility, and they should probably not be living on their own in any case.

Keep a list of all medications in your wallet or purse for emergencies. It becomes a back-up for your medical folder.

If the name of the medicine or the directions for use are not easy to read or understand as printed on the container, ask the pharmacist to make the print larger, or give you more verbal information or provide an information sheet. You are not being a nuisance: this is what they are trained for – to provide the best service to maintain people's health.

Other health concerns

Be observant of, and sensitive to, your charge's general health and possible ailments other than those of dementia: they may not be able to tell you about their aches and pains, and you have to be observant. If they are quieter or rowdier than usual, they may have wax in their ears or in their hearing aid; or they may be developing a virus and starting to feel rotten. Sometimes changes that appear to have a medical basis do not, but it is good to get them checked out anyway.

Watching out for strokes

If the person you are caring for is developing vascular dementia, you and your doctor need to be aware of their blood pressure and incipient transient ischaemic attacks (TIAs). Doctors can treat strokes and help reduce the risk of future strokes successfully – if they start treatment within three hours (the sooner the better: immediately is best).

Signs of another stroke can include:

- sudden weakness, numbness or paralysis of face, arm or leg, especially on one side of the body
- sudden blurred or dimmed vision, especially in one eye, or an episode of double vision
- difficulty speaking or understanding even simple sentences
- dizziness or loss of balance or coordination, especially when combined with another symptom
- a sudden, unexplained and intense headache
- sudden nausea and fever – distinguished from a viral illness by the speed of onset (minutes or hours rather than days)
- brief loss of consciousness or a period of decreased awareness (fainting, confusion, convulsions, coma).

Sometimes these signs may appear for a very short period of time and then disappear. Do not ignore them, as they may indicate serious stroke risks,

and a full stroke may follow. For a quick test ask the person to:
1. raise both arms
2. poke out their tongue
3. smile
4. say a sentence.

If they can't do these simple tasks after an 'incident', phone immediately for the ambulance.

After a fall

Some dementias, such as LBD, make falls more likely. If your charge falls, don't hurry to get them on their feet again. First make sure they have not injured themselves. Then ask them whether they want to get up. If not, put a cushion under their head, cover them with a rug and leave them until they are ready to make a move.

When they are ready, avoid straining yourself trying to lift them.
1. Pull a chair, or some stable, low article of furniture, close to them and help them get on their hands and knees.
2. Support them as they put one hand on the chair seat, and help them to raise one leg so that the foot is flat on the ground with the knee bent.
3. Put your hands around their waist (or put one shoulder under their chest) to support them as they put weight onto the foot flat on the ground, put both their hands on the chair and bring up the other foot so they are sort of squatting.
4. They should now be able, still with support, to push up with their legs, stand up and, possibly, sit on the chair for a breather.

Use your medical alarm, if you have one, or phone the local fire brigade or ambulance branch if you need help with a lift. If you are really concerned, call the emergency services number.

Checking for dehydration

People with dementia, the elderly and those in nursing homes are especially vulnerable to dehydration. It can be serious, but its symptoms – such as flushing, rapid pulse, dizziness, confusion, vomiting – are easily confused with other problems.

Two initial ways to check for dehydration are to see if the person's urine is dark, which can indicate dehydration, and to do the 'pinch test'. This test involves grasping a piece of skin (often the back of the hand, but in an elderly person, the forehead or breastbone is better), holding for several seconds, then letting go. Skin with normal elasticity returns to its usual position quickly, but with decreased elasticity it returns slowly. The latter, too, can indicate dehydration. The pinch test need not hurt.

If in doubt, always check with a doctor or nurse. Dehydration is easily treated. (See also Chapter 19: Eating and Drinking, 'Getting enough fluids'.)

Drowsiness or sleeplessness

If the person with dementia spends a lot of time snoozing, check that they aren't becoming ill. Drowsiness is not a symptom you should expect – usually just the opposite.

A high percentage of adults complain about not getting a good night's sleep, but the problem is even more widespread among people with dementia. Check to see whether the following could be responsible and try making adjustments:

- too much coffee, tea or alcohol
- agitation caused by upset with you, their carer, or others
- strange environment, disturbing shadows
- too early to bed, too many naps during the day, or not enough exercise
- hunger or thirst, being too hot or cold.

If you can rule those out, report to your doctor in case the sleeplessness is caused by:

- infections
- an additional illness, such as angina, diabetes or ulcers
- pain from conditions such as arthritis, strains or gout
- side-effects of medications
- stress or depression.

In an experiment, some Alzheimer's patients with sleeping problems spent two-hour periods during the day in front of bright panels, while others simply had brighter light bulbs placed in their living rooms. Compared with a control group, both groups showed improvement in their sleep patterns and body temperature. Outdoor sunlight and exercise also appeared to help.

Natural therapies

You may wish to try other ways of boosting the health of the person you are looking after and making life easier for them. Complementary therapies do not tackle the cause of the dementia or delay its progress, but may still benefit patients and carers. Your charge may find touch and personal care soothing, with agitation and sleep disturbances lessening; while you as their carer may feel less stress and be able to relax better.

Always inform your doctor of what you are doing, and go to a qualified and recommended practitioner of the complementary therapy. Doctors may even have these alternative skills themselves. (See also 'Medical breakthroughs and natural wonders', above.)

Reflexology

It is claimed that, by massaging reflex areas in the feet that correspond to parts of the body, the therapist stimulates energy and readjustment to the out-of-balance body. This technique is promoted for stress and tension reduction.

Psychotherapy

Sessions of psychotherapy can pinpoint life problems that contribute to depression. Using types such as cognitive therapy can help explore negative or distorted patterns of thinking and behaving that contribute to feelings of despair and helplessness.

Psychotherapists can also help their clients to understand which aspects of the problems can be solved or improved, identify realistic goals for improving emotional well-being, and regain a sense of control and pleasure in life.

It is questionable whether psychotherapy can really be helpful for people with dementia. Certainly it may help you in your caring role.

Nutritional therapy

This uses special diets and food supplements to prevent and treat disease; but dietary changes of this nature should be made only in consultation with your doctor.

For instance, cranberry capsules are promoted for people who are prone to urinary tract infections – including those with dementia, who can be reluctant to drink and thus have insufficient fluids to flush out the bladder. Dispensing of medication for urinary tract infections to one hospital's residents was reportedly reduced after they began taking the capsules. However, cranberry may thin the blood, so you should be cautious about using it at the same time as medically prescribed anticoagulants.

Herbalism

Remedies are claimed to restore balance to the body and help it to heal itself. For instance, an extract from leaves of the Ginkgo biloba tree is said to stimulate circulation and increase the flow of oxygen to the brain, and, although several clinical trials have shown the use of this extract to be ineffective in the treatment of dementia, remedies such as this can have a helpful placebo effect.

Massage

Probably the oldest and simplest form of health care, this is based on the healing value of touch. Massage can soothe and relax, release muscle tension and improve circulation.

Homeopathy

This uses the 'like cures like' principle. A substance that can cause similar symptoms to the illness being treated is used, in an extremely diluted form, to stimulate the body's healing capacity. Research evidence is slim, but certainly some people report they have benefited.

Acupuncture

This technique from traditional Chinese medicine is based on the theory that energy (or chi) flows through pathways (meridians) in the body.

Maintaining Health

The practitioner inserts needles into the skin at specific points to restore and balance the flow of energy. Acupuncture can be beneficial for stress, insomnia and pain relief, and to relax muscles. Users of the technique range from Chinese medicine practitioners to some physiotherapists.

Aromatherapy

Plant extracts, in the form of very concentrated oils, can be added to a hot bath, used with massage, applied in compresses, or placed on a tissue and inhaled. They are particularly beneficial in relieving stress, anxiety, insomnia and depression.

Where to from here

- Chapter 3: Understanding Dementia
- Chapter 7: Dealing with Health Professionals
- Chapter 8: Adapting the Home Environment, especially 'First aid kit'
- Chapter 16: Exercise
- Chapter 19: Eating and Drinking
- Chapter 20: Showering and Dressing
- Chapter 21: Toileting
- Chapter 23: Hallucinations, Delusions and Delirium, especially 'Delirium'

Chapter 16

Exercise

Benefits

Exercise benefits both carers and those cared for. Physically, it boosts strength (something carers use every day) and maintains flexibility, coordination and balance (to reduce risks of falls and fractures). It boosts circulation, promotes regular bladder and bowel functions, develops healthy appetites and leads to increased energy.

Other benefits of exercise are that it burns up adrenalin (a hormone produced by stress and frustration), and produces endorphins (hormones that promote relaxation and well-being). It improves mood and sleep, and helps prevent the dementia-related agitation and restlessness known as sundowning (Chapter 9: Managing Difficult Behaviour, 'Sundowning or twilighting').

When it is familiar and a routine, exercise also calms the body and mind, and if done outdoors or with others gives both you and your charge a sense of belonging in the community. Doing it together can cement the relationship between you and become something special you share.

> Connie used to walk with Trevor most afternoons. They went very slowly as far as he could manage with his walker, which was 200 metres along their road. At that point they would sit on a seat outside the local dairy for 20 minutes or so. This break, watching the world go by, gave Connie practice in patience and Trevor strength for the homeward journey. It also created a bunch of new acquaintances from among the dairy's customers.

> Once home again, while he could still be safely left on his own, Connie would settle Trevor in his chair with his radio, then leave for her own walk. The first time, she puffed so badly that she could hardly make it up the first steep rise. After a couple of weeks, however, she was fitter, strode up that slope easily and began walking further. It did wonders for her physical and mental health.

Crucially, physical activity helps someone with dementia to be independent for longer. If your doctor or specialist says it would be beneficial, go for it. Make it a regular commitment for as long as possible.

Reluctant or unable?

Exercise can seem a big demand for a carer who is already exhausted by anxiety, patience and the sheer effort of every day's tasks and goes to bed very tired each night. It can also be frustrating, when the activity involved is very slow, minimal and confined. Your charge may also be unwilling to use their limited energy on the extra effort required or they may not be motivated to exercise on their own.

> Gina wanted to do her very best for Bert. Though his movements were fairly limited by now, she thought that they could do a daily exercise routine together, following notes and diagrams left by the visiting physio.
>
> She stopped after a week. 'All very well for physios,' she grumped, 'they get paid; but I'm his wife. I'm not paid and I just don't have 30 or 40 minutes every morning to do those b___ exercises. Bert just has to motivate himself.'
>
> Unfortunately Bert stopped those exercises too, wouldn't go to a course of physio classes, said the local rehabilitation hospital's swimming pool was unsuitable for walking in, and was too fastidious to go to the public heated pool.

Researchers are beginning to understand that the motivational area of the brain can be affected in people with dementia. The person does not seem guilty or regretful about it, and doesn't worry that they sit around a lot, while a carer may assume they are being lazy, giving up, or just being difficult. Nevertheless, 'use it or lose it' applies to everyone, and both of you will benefit from regularly using limbs and muscles and getting the heart pumping harder.

When your charge is tired, they may sometimes imagine pain, complain of it and try to avoid physical activity. You may have heard of this psychological effect and jolly them along. But take care: their pain may not necessarily be in the mind. Note their comments about pain or dizziness or shortness of breath and act on them. The symptoms may not be related to dementia but to some other health problem. Consult a doctor if the person mentions something out of the ordinary.

Other factors that may affect the ability or willingness to exercise are:
- over-medication, especially when sedatives are used (see Chapter 15: Maintaining Health, 'Cautionary notes')
- worsening motor symptoms, where the spirit and mind are willing but the body is weak.

A normal person who continues exercise when tired builds up further stamina. A person with dementia who continues exercise when tired (especially if they have Parkinson's or Lewy body dementias) is more likely to fall. So don't let the person with dementia feel guilty about resting during the day, or limiting their exercise. Their disability takes much strength out of them. They need to recuperate. Don't nag, either – but do note that sometimes encouragement is useful, because losing too much function may threaten the affected person's wish to be cared for at home.

This is another challenge for you – keeping a sensible balance. One person with dementia has expressed it like this:

> Let us sit and doze or gaze into space without feeling guilty, but keep us going with irregular interruptions of snacks or stimulation or exercise.

Looking at options

If the person you are caring for is motivated, let them choose their exercise and do it as much as possible. Try to offer purpose for the workout, keep everything fun, and laugh.

Dancing of any sort is a great way to use energy, have enjoyment and produce a good night's sleep. Alternatively, you could explore the physiotherapy classes offered for those with dementia. If physiotherapy classes don't appeal, find out about other activities from the local senior citizens' centre. Your charge will probably try anything they suggest, if you go too. Group activities aren't for everybody.

Home exercises might be preferable, and if no one else is able to be present in person, a DVD, television exercise programme or even a console game (such as Wii Fit) might do the trick.

Getting started

+ They should wear loose clothes (appropriate for the temperature) with pants elasticated around the waist and ankles, and shoes with Velcro straps. Remember they can forget to put on or take off clothes as they get cold or hot, so do it for them.
+ Use familiar warm-ups and make them fun. For instance, pretending to be athletes, walk up and down, or march on the spot for a few minutes. Stretch the upper and lower body and limbs gently. Reach to pick non-existent apples high up in a tree, or from the ground. Use your imagination.

Walking

This is the easiest and most accessible form of exercise for your charge on their own (if they won't get lost) or both of you together. You will both work out how far and fast you can go. Walk together regularly, at the same time and on the same route if possible.

If they have Parkinson's, encourage them to:
+ put their heel down first on each step
+ move forward on to their toe (otherwise they tend to walk on tip-toe)
+ swing their arms
+ take frequent rests (to reset their mind to walking, not running, mode)
+ walk once a day at least without tiring themselves.

They may have trouble remembering these hints for walking, but some may catch on.

Chapter 16

One man with Lewy body dementia was determined to keep himself in shape:

> After he had been diagnosed with LBD, Arthur exercised by himself as often as possible. This included walking their poodle to the park for the first five years. After the dog died, however, Arthur's walk gradually became a shuffle and his walking distance reduced. He adopted a walking stick, and later a walking frame.
>
> By then he could just make it to the top of his road and back each day. He felt a bit scared, because coming home was slightly downhill and he knew he might start running if he wasn't careful, so he gripped his walker's hand-brake levers all the way home. This actually stopped the wheels going round at all and ground down their rubber tyres.
>
> He finished up with square wheels, which made a distinctive 'clunk, clunk, clunk'. Everyone knew when Arthur was coming. The hospital's fixers were incredibly understanding and non-judgemental as they replaced the tyres regularly.

Tips for walking

- Try walking in twos with another couple. This gives the carer a chance to unload a little, while another person chats to your charge.
- Find a scented garden to explore; or wade in waist-high warm water at a local pool.
- Go to different eating places for a drink or lunch (outside, so no worry about crumbs) and park your car a good walk away.
- Ask your charge to push the supermarket trolley. Carry a bag and shopping list and, perhaps, give them the money so they feel independent. But choose the time and place carefully: busy shopping centres can be exhausting and stressful, with diverse loud noises from all directions.
- If they use a wheelchair sometimes, and ask to push you for a change, let them have a go.
- Visit an orchard to pick fruit. Take a folding chair in case they get tired.

- If it is raining, walk anywhere covered and interesting: zoo, bird sanctuary, museums, art galleries, and especially 'old time' exhibitions.
- Walk along suburban streets and decide which houses you'd like to live in and why.
- Walk a dog or push a grandchild in a stroller.

Using walking aids

Your occupational therapist can provide your charge with a walking frame. Some people are reluctant to use one initially, but the right encouragement will help. It will improve their mobility significantly.

> Gary, unwilling to be seen using a walker, was sitting rather forlornly at a funeral wake one morning when two women he knew came up to him. They were both using walkers, and were moving with confidence among the assembled mourners. One of them said, 'Gary, you should get one of these. How do you like my new one? It's such a lovely red. I call it my Ferrari!'

Brightly coloured models are available with trays in front (for cups of tea or glasses of beer), baskets underneath for the shopping, and a seat for rests. You may even be able to make sensible additions yourself, using common household equipment, to make it is as good – and as safe – as it can be for you and your charge.

> One day, when Bill walked too far for his own good, Joss sat him on his walker's seat and pushed him home. But his legs weren't strong enough to hold his feet off the ground and he wore large holes in his trousers, where they flopped under his shoes dragging on the pavement.
>
> To avoid a repeat, Joss took her empty peg apron when they went walking. If Bill tired, she would sit him on his walker's seat facing her, tie the peg apron round her waist, lift his legs and tuck his shoe heels into the loose pockets of the apron and they could get along fine. She didn't mind how Bill looked all folded up, and he was relieved to be pushed when he was exhausted.

A walker gives good (although not infallible) stability, but they may let it get further and further in front of them until they are at full stretch and starting to run. Something soft and wide, attached to each handle and placed round their buttocks, can help to prevent this.

To stop Bruce running, Alison bought two strong elastic bungee cords with hooks at each end. She positioned Bruce ready to walk with the walking frame, slipped one hook of each elastic cord into the right handle of the walker, stretched one cord across his back at waist height and fixed its other hook into the left handle, then pulled the other cord under his bottom and hooked it into the same handle.

Bruce said he felt embarrassed and rather like a racehorse in a crupper after he was fitted up, but the harness kept him close to the frame and stopped his running.

Exercises

The following exercises keep your charge's muscles in trim for moving in different directions. These variations on the walking theme will suit some people, but should be undertaken only with the ready consent of your charge. Do them to music.

Obtain two pieces of dowelling, about 1.5 metres long. Wrap sticky tape round each end. These become handles.

Forwards walk

1. Stand behind your charge in a spacious area with a smooth and level surface, such as a hall or driveway.
2. Put one handle of each stick in their right and left hands. Hold the other handles yourself, in your matching right and left hands, parallel to the floor.
3. Say, 'Let's practise swinging them,' and the two of you swing them back and forth.
4. Then say, 'We're going to march and these will help. Are you ready? Now, beginning with your left foot, left, right, left, right…' and you march off, swinging the arms (and sticks) forwards and backwards, just as you would if you were marching.

5. Walk maybe 40 paces forwards, turn around and return to starting point.
6. Repeat once, if they are keen.

Backwards walk

This is less easy, but a nice challenge. Be careful.
1. Stand behind your charge, where you can watch their balance.
2. Tell them you are both going to walk backwards slowly, swinging the sticks
3. Suggest they keep legs well apart so they don't tangle them up.
4. Do 20 of these.
5. March forward again to the start.
6. Repeat, if they are keen.

For a more advanced version of these exercises, stand behind your charge without the sticks and suggest they try a similar forwards and backwards walk, with you there to guide and help. Be ready with a steadying hand.

Sideways walk

1. Stand facing your charge, holding a dowelling stick between you in each hand.
2. Say, 'Now we are going to take sideways steps to your right.'
3. Take one step sideways with your left foot (remember, you are a mirror image to the other person), and bring your right foot up beside it.
4. Repeat 10 or 15 times.
5. Reverse the direction and return to where you started.

More help for people with LBD and PDD

Place strips of visible sticky tape or foot outlines on hallways, and other often-used walking areas outside. Space these 'stepping stones' at a distance comfortable for your charge. With a bit of concentration by them, this helps walking and reduces 'freezing' episodes.

If your charge freezes and forgets how to put one foot in front of the other, put one of your feet (or a torch spotlight, or an object) on the floor in front of them. Ask them to step over it, making sure that you have a

steadying hand available at all times. An alternative is to suggest that the person:
- ✦ visualises an imaginary object on the floor to step over
- ✦ looks at an object ahead and walks to it
- ✦ counts in a regular rhythmic voice and walks to the rhythm.

If they can't start, suggest they place their feet wide apart and rock from side to side, or march in place, then take off when the time seems right.

Another potential aid for someone who has 'frozen' is a metronome, ticking to give them a sense of the rhythm of walking.

When your person with dementia 'freezes' regularly, you may need to keep a collapsible wheelchair in the car.

Exercise after a stroke

If the person you are caring for is left with only moderate dementia after a stroke, you could both start:
- ✦ 20–60 minutes of walking or similar exercise (may be done in two or three spells) three to seven days a week
- ✦ flying a kite
- ✦ strength training, using weights or resistance; 10–15 repetitions two or three times a week – do 8–10 different exercises working the legs, arms, back and other muscle groups
- ✦ balance or coordination exercises 2–3 times a week.

In or on the water

If your charge is a long-time sailor who can no longer sail on their own, they may appreciate it if you go with them. It's best in a gentle breeze when there is no chance of tipping over.

Swimming is one of the best all-round exercises. The feeling of being in a warm pool can be very soothing and calming. For some, a previous fear of drowning is no longer a problem:

> One woman learned to swim when she was in the middle stages of dementia. She forgot that she'd always been afraid of water!

Generally, though, the person needs to be comfortable and confident in the water – and a cautious start is a good idea.

Sybil had been an active woman, but these days she stooped and dragged on Paul's arm when walking or had to use a walker. 'Why don't you both go "water jogging"?' suggested a friend. 'It's been my saviour. Come tomorrow and I'll show you.'

Wearing their swimsuits, Paul and Sybil met her at the pool and watched her put on a simple flotation harness. She entered the deep end and began 'walking' through the water. It looked very simple and Sybil, though not a good swimmer, said she would give it a go.

So Paul put a harness on them both and practised on his own before helping Sybil in. She clutched him and the railing tightly. 'Come on, bean bag,' he said cheerfully. 'It's magical. You'll be okay,' and he pulled her away from the railing and set off, holding one of her hands.

Sybil shrieked and grabbed him, pushing him underwater. The flotation harness had made her legs float up behind her and her face go under. Paul surfaced spluttering and hauled her upright. He felt he might still drown as he pushed her, scrabbling all over him, some metres back to safety. He cursed himself for not letting her hold the railing.

Ball games

Versions of familiar ball games can be enjoyable. For soccer, kick a ball, or something softer, into a makeshift goal (say, between two shrubs) rather than trying to dribble it, which may cause falls. Rugby can be as simple as tossing a rugby ball between you both.

Tennis can involve a tennis ball against a volley board, either with a racquet or just thrown and caught. Another ball game for two or more, perhaps including the grandchildren, is to bat a balloon around, keeping it in the air. For easier golfing, buy a small-mesh net and set it up for them to drive golf balls into – from not too far away.

Bowls may also be popular with some.

Five or six years into his LBD, Alan enjoyed going to bowls for a short roll-up, so long as it was just with Judy. He hated someone else joining them.

He had been a handy bowler and could still put bowls round the jack, but within six months he sometimes bowled on the wrong bias. He couldn't work out which way to hold the bowl, so Judy put a white sticker on each bowl's bias side. This helped for a few months until he didn't want to go bowling at all.

They continued walking together, however; and he kept on playing golf with Judy, his brother and one or two understanding old friends, scoring his first ever hole-in-one.

The important thing is to exercise according to your charge's capabilities, adapting an existing game as appropriate, and moving on to another as abilities change.

Seated exercises

Both of you can do these exercises in straight-backed chairs, facing each other. Have regular rest periods.

Kick the ball (no ball included!)

Lift one foot, straighten that leg then return it to the floor. Do this five times to start, then 10 times, either alternating legs or several with one leg then several with the other. The quadriceps muscles on the upper thighs may get a little stiff as a result. After a few days, and when they are no longer stiff, increase the number of lifts. After weeks of improvement, strap a 500-gram weight to the ankle.

Sit and march

Take high steps, raising knees – left, right, left, right – 10 times. Again, muscles may rebel at first, but should improve with practice, and you may feel you can 'march' for miles.

Kick my hand

Your charge sits on the chair. You sit or crouch in front and hold your hand 30 centimetres or so above the floor and ask them to kick it (great for angry people). Check with them, lowering or raising your hand as you see fit and to meet their abilities.

Other physical activities

Even outdoor tasks are a form of exercise. Your charge could paint a fence with stain (not as difficult as with paint, but do lay a protective sheet to catch drips). They could also dig or hoe an unspoilable part of the garden.

Gentle gym workouts are another option, while physiotherapy, Alexander technique, yoga, or tai chi are all good for a person with only moderate dementia. Try a mixture, which will bring interest and motivation, but balance it with routine. Tai chi is a more sociable form of exercise, although it involves more brain work.

> Connie discovered tai chi later, and she and Trevor went together.
> Trevor did his tai chi sitting in a chair. Connie did hers with the main group.

Where to from here

✦ Chapter 9: Managing Difficult Behaviour
✦ Chapter 10: Wider Support and Self-care, 'Quick recuperation for carers'
✦ Chapter 11: Independence and Safety
✦ Chapter 15: Maintaining Health
✦ Chapter 17: Entertainment
✦ Chapter 18: Holidays and Travel, 'Exercises for both of you on a plane'
✦ Chapter 21: Toileting

Chapter 17

Entertainment

Dementia affects people in widely differing ways: some sit for long periods quietly dozing and staring into space (making you wonder if they need stimulation), some are frenetically active, or repeat the same question over and over, or follow you around constantly. Sometimes you feel like exploding.

> Helen had never been able to relax in her and Donald's old home. He fell often on the steeply sloping section, and he would take off walking, often losing his way, or stopping the traffic while he ambled across the busy road.
>
> At their new apartment, she still could not relax – Donald was never more than a metre away from her. He felt totally lost in the strange environment, and wanted to be with her and know what she was doing every minute of every day.

Most people affected by dementia are somewhere in between. Some of the activities here – or variations that you may come up with – should suit your charge, improve the way you both spend your hours, and help strengthen your relationship if you do them together. Build up a list of activities they can do, inside and out, and share these with your support group.

> Stephen did his best to look after his partner, Olwyn, now in her early seventies. She had developed vascular dementia. At times, when he thought she was looking vacant too long, he would sit with her at their kitchen table and start her polishing the brass fire irons and horse brasses she had inherited from her old family home.

If the person is in care

If the person with dementia is in care, you may wish to include others at the home in your activities. Add to the library (DVDs, large-print books and talking books, especially those of yesteryear); or play music, CDs or DVDs to a group. Spend time talking to residents, too: as they get to know you, they will respond and light up when they see you. Otherwise you could simply sit with your charge during home entertainment, and take them for a special walk outside. (See Chapter 10: Wider Support and Self-care, 'From a distance', for suggestions about how an out-of-town family member can help with entertainments.)

Regular activity

Being active makes life seem normal, helps the person you are caring for maintain their skills, and keeps them alert and interested in people and happenings. It can also be fun!

Wherever your charge is on the behaviour scale, they need some daily activity; it can be anything that might hold their attention. They are happiest with familiar routines.

> Doug would vacuum the car for Gloria, and check oil and water and tyre pressure, long after he could no longer drive.

They can even enjoy doing nothing, if they are with you. However, for your sanity and so that you can get things done as 'sole runner of the household', have a range of potential activities available.

Encouraging your charge
Participation, not perfection

The person you are looking after doesn't want to be 'cared for' all the time. They need a sense of involvement and achievement, and to be doing simple tasks as they used to. This can make them feel good, providing they see the tasks as being of value. It doesn't matter if the job is not well done, so long as they feel they've achieved something.

> Alan used to set the table when he and Judy had people in for a meal. Now he still set it, but the mats, cutlery and glasses would be placed higgledy-piggledy and the napkins in an untidy pile in

the middle. Once he even put the table mats on the carpet under the table with the cutlery in heaps on top of them, something she opted to remedy! But he remained happy to do the job – and she continued to ask him.

If your charge doesn't finish what they're doing, you can – after you have praised them and they have moved off.

Boosting motivation

Dementia affects people's motivation, so help them get started. Stop the activity if they look like becoming frustrated, bored or upset because they are unable to finish what they have begun. Ask if they'd like help, or just let it lapse without comment and finish it yourself.

Be positive without being bossy, and don't get downhearted if the person with dementia is unenthusiastic. Accept 'No, I don't want to' cheerfully. It's not entertainment if it's not voluntary. If they have been 'making themselves useful', thank them and say how helpful they've been.

Activities you suggest should be safe yet stimulating, without too many challenges or choices, as these can lead to behavioural problems. They should ideally be familiar and based on previous skills, hobbies and occupations, so your charge can feel successful even if they are slow. If numbers or reading cause problems, leave them out, and if they get mad at their loss of skill, it's probably better that they watch instead. A few new activities can be suitable, providing they are easy enough not to be confusing. Some entertainments may fill only one to five minutes. Others may fill one or two hours, especially if you are away from home. Try to alternate shorter and longer activities, and to organise activities that can be done in short bursts.

If they find it difficult to choose what to do and end up doing nothing, that's okay. Since you can't be everything and everyone to them, look around for family, friends or community centres to assist with diversions.

Entertainments based on previous occupations

You might like to put a small tick in the margin beside each activity below when you use it, and add a mark out of 10 as to how successful it was.

Art

Place a solid easel, and paper sheets held by bulldog clips, on a wide plastic protector sheet. Put out jars of water-based blue, yellow, red and black paints on a stand, and a large white board or plate to mix colours on. Have easy-to-hold paint brushes, a water jar for rinsing, and a space where the finished works can lie.

Alternatively, buy charcoal to use instead of paints. Remember that great effects can be obtained by smudging the lines. Or let the person you are caring for experiment with pencil or crayon sketching and stencils, probably best on a flat table surface.

Cards

Given a card table and a pack of cards, your charge may try a game of simple patience, or just shuffle the cards around and deal hands of sorts.

> One couple played contract bridge every Wednesday night with friends, who said they wanted to carry on after Hermione's Alzheimer's diagnosis. She could still bid and play cards. Then she started to forget what trumps were, so with their friends' approval her husband glued a card from a different suit onto the sides of a light bulb cardboard box (which was just the right size), and wrote 'No Trumps' on the top. As they played each hand, he turned the box so Hermione could see what trumps were. They went on playing for quite a while.

Cooking

Your charge can help prepare a meal (even if only one potato is peeled) and set the table. If you are baking, they can help sift dry ingredients, butter pans, or cream butter and sugar with a wooden spoon. Making pikelets is easy.

They retain their sense of taste, touch, smell and hearing when concentration and reasoning disappear, so try a 'tasting for memories' experience. Let them sit and sample different dishes, or cakes or biscuits, when they are fresh from the oven. Sweet, sour, crisp, soft, flaky, chewy, cold or hot – each one should evoke pleasure, interest or memories you can share.

Ray was a chocaholic, and he had never let Peggy forget his mother's home-baked chocolate cookies. So, as his dementia deepened, she often bought chocolate cookies for his snacks, and served up chocolate blancmange (still warm) with his ice cream. When she jogged his memory, he sometimes reminisced about his youth. She would be bored because she knew it all after 40 years together, but occasionally she would sit up in surprise, when he came out with something she'd never heard before.

Dressmaking or fashion

Set out plain and graph paper and coloured pencils or felt pens for designing. Assemble a pile of women's fashion magazines to thumb through.

Caroline had worked all her life in clothing manufacture. When dementia took over in her late sixties, her head still turned in the street if she saw a well-dressed person, and she liked to push her walker to the shops, where she could spend 10 minutes admiring the display in the window of a smart women's clothing boutique.

Fishing

An old angler may like to finger the flies in their fly fishing case; or cast a line on the back lawn. The hook on the fly can be cut back to the shank to avoid hurting themselves or anyone else.

Gardening

Inside or out, your companion could repot plants. Having material just out of reach will encourage stretching, which is also good for the body. Enable them to grow something by putting a bulb, cut carrot or turnip top on pebbles covered by water in a shallow dish. Keep it in a light place and watch it sprout.

Outside, using dishwasher detergent and wire twisted into a loop, encourage the person you are looking after to blow bubbles and watch where they go. They could also sit in the garden, resting their tired feet in a foot spa of warm water. Or, as an outing, visit a scented garden. These, created with blind people in mind, are located at botanic gardens or other public places.

As you prune trees, they can cut the prunings into smaller lengths. They may injure themselves a bit sometimes, but a bandaged finger may be worth it. Raking fallen leaves off paths and lawns or watering the garden are other outdoor occupations involving good use of muscles.

Golf
Keep clubs, and a few old golf balls in a bag, for an occasional swing (without a ball) or a few chip shots on the lawn – or for pottering around a putting green. Buy light plastic 'skeleton' balls for full-blooded drives which go almost nowhere.

Home care
Activities include cleaning flower pots, or washing the car or the outside windows with a long-handled sponge. They could clean windows with crumpled newspaper and methylated spirits or turpentine or just plain water. Your charge might also clean the front and back doors and windowsills.

Ironing – with the temperature gauge set at warm (not hot) – is another possibility, and later on they could fold or hang the pressed clothes. They could fold dry laundry such as towels, and put socks into pairs.

Other tasks include watering pot plants, mopping the floor, dusting, putting away unbreakable items, feeding the birds and collecting the mail.

Music and dance
The person you are looking after may enjoy listening to a radio with simple controls tuned to a favourite radio station. Perhaps have one by their bed, another by a most-used armchair. If music comes on, give them:
- a baton (pencil?) to conduct with and space to dance in
- rice in a lidded tin container to shake in time, Spanish castanets to click
- a drum or triangle to play.

It helps if someone else plays a musical instrument as well.

Fill glasses or bottles with varying levels of water to make a scale or just a variety of notes when tapped with a knife. CDs of old songs can be a wonderful resource at your local library. Your charge can dance and sing to some of these old tunes. If you have the opportunity to take them to hear live music and see the players or singers, this may prove even more rewarding.

> One very demented patient, who had played a wind instrument for years, was now in the secure unit of a retirement home. Although her family tried to keep her interest up with CDs, tapes and the radio, she just waved them away; but when her old orchestra gave a concert in the home's lounge she was rapt, moved with the music and seemed more settled for a while after.

Mute, isolated individuals will sometimes respond to music.

> Alison, having joined Bruce at day care for the Christmas sing-along, sat with him at a table with four other silent, hunched-over men, who stared into space and didn't take part. After a few songs, one of them pointed to her song book, leant over and began to sing as she shared it.

Office work

For an ex-office worker or professional, leave a few books lying around; but don't push them – your charge may get frustrated because they've 'lost it'. Supply stationery items such as A4 paper (reuse sheets printed on only one side), a stapler, a hole punch, a ring binder, pencils rather than messy ballpoint pens, a ruler, a ledger-type exercise book, paper clips, and so on. These items, spread out on a special work table or desk (ideally with a drawer or three), may have them 'keeping the accounts up to date' for hours.

> Carol, formerly a high-powered accountant in a city firm, developed dementia in her early seventies. A relative went to a second-hand dealer, paid $25 for an old desk and waste paper tin, and set them up in Carol's living room. With a plentiful supply of office paraphernalia at hand, her time was filled to everyone's contentment.

Toolshed tasks

Collect nuts and bolts to be matched up and screwed together, hammer and nails, a brace and bit, screws and screwdriver and blocks of softish wood to work on.

If you obtain an old car door from the wrecker's yard, your charge might be kept happy for quite some time hammering out the dents.

They might be able to oil and even sharpen garden tools. For a less able person, make power tools available to handle (not turned on), or put a box of old tools out to explore.

> Even when he got Alzheimer's, Alex always kept busy making blocks as gifts for his great-grandchildren. He sanded smooth cubes of wood that his son cut from wood off-cuts, and painted them with food colourings. When they dried, he boxed them in sets of different colours and shapes, wrapped them and tied them with ribbon. His son had to write the card, though.

Inside occupations
Television, DVDs, radio and films

The most popular television for people with dementia includes wildlife, gardening and home-care shows. Find out what your charge likes best, but be aware they may be content spending long periods just gazing at anything on the screen.

> Blair's son gave his ex-All Black father the Rugby Channel for a month's trial as a Christmas gift. Blair had had Parkinson's dementia for four years and his son knew he spent a lot of time sitting in front of the television. But in fact Blair watched any subject on television for 10 minutes at the most. After that he was just staring into space.

Try some of the older, well-known comedies available on DVD, or listen to the news on radio or television and talk about it.

People with dementia will probably not sit through a full-length film or play at a theatre, but even if you leave partway through, they may have enjoyed the outing.

> Elaine and Sweeney thought they would like to see the latest *Lord of the Rings* film, but felt he could not last its nearly four hours. They

explained this to the cinema's manager, and he reserved the same two seats for them on consecutive days. 'You'll have to find them in the dark on the second day,' he commented, asking if she thought they'd be able to. 'We'll make sure we can,' Elaine replied, then she and Sweeney paid and went in.

They saw the whole film on the one day. Sweeney wasn't restive; they were both enthralled. 'You did so well, darling. What a compliment to Peter Jackson,' Elaine said to Sweeney as they came out. 'Do you think we should write and tell him?' Sweeney was too exhausted to reply, but he talked about the film enthusiastically during the next few days.

Armchair activities at home

Turn the pages of newspapers, magazines and old school journals. Even if the person you are caring for can't read, the pictures occupy their attention: they will go through them again and again. Read from the newspaper, a book of familiar poems, the Bible or a favourite story, and see how they react.

Ask them to say their favourite word of the moment, then discuss it. Attempt an easy crossword or word puzzles from the newspaper or inexpensive collections of puzzles.

> Lindsay continued to be entertained and energised by the word puzzles that his wife Jane brought him. His speech was almost incomprehensible, and he recognised few of his friends, but he could still pick out words in a grid of letters and loved to settle to the task. Jane found herself stretched to keep up a supply for him until she realised he didn't remember the ones he'd done before. She began photocopying each puzzle dozens of times.

Talk about what you've been doing, leaving generous silences for their reactions (this is more productive than asking them questions).

Check your local library's collection of talking books for anything suitable. Look at holiday diaries, letters and pamphlets of countries visited. Bring out old photo albums and go through them.

They may also like to cut out paper pictures with scissors (with rounded ends), or sort buttons and/or wool. Another craft possibility is using a blunt embroidery needle to sew on an old tea towel or piece of suitable plain material, following an outlined pattern or stencil. They could also knit squares for patchwork blankets.

They might like to cuddle a doll or soft toy, to fondle gentle and patient household pets – a cat or rabbit in the lap, a dog at the feet – or to play with a kitten and a piece of paper tied to string. This is all good exercise for the hands. So is squashing a soft rubber ball.

At a table

Cover a table with easily cleaned material, and provide a long-keeping 'playdough' to knead or mould. This is easily made: sift 2 cups plain flour, ½ cup salt and 2 tablespoons cream of tartar. Add 2 tablespoons cooking oil, 2 cups boiling water and (optional) 1 teaspoon food colouring. Mix well, form a clump and store in an airtight container until needed.

Endless occupation can be had with this, using just a rolling pin, shaped biscuit-cutters or their hands and fingers. Alternatively, obtain or buy large lumps of clay and exercise the hands by working it into usable consistency, after which you can both sit and make whatever comes into your head. Suggest worms and snakes, snakes coiled into pots or jars, little animals, or models of each other.

Play solitaire, dominoes, draughts, Chinese chequers, housie, or snakes and ladders, changing the rules as required. Another option is to play marbles on a table cloth – rolling along lines, knocking others away – like indoor bowls.

The person you look after may be happy drawing, cutting out, or doing collage (perhaps with coloured leaves). Keep materials handy for making a scrapbook: newsprint, A4 sheets of paper with blank backs, half-used pads, exercise books, glossy magazines; or more sophisticated papers, stickers and so on from a 'scrapbooking' hobby store. Use coloured pens and pencils; round-ended scissors; paste or glue.

They could also make a photo album using an exercise book, glue, old photos and a 'naming' pen. Consider starting a family tree for them, and extend their life book (see Chapter 6: Becoming a Carer, 'Life book').

Write down the stories they tell you. The interest shown by you or a grandchild may be much appreciated, if this wistful comment from a person with dementia is anything to go by:

> It would be great if you would learn a bit more about the local, national and world history of my youth. My recent memory cells may have shrivelled and died, but my old memories can be revived and relived and ... I may even teach you a thing or two!

Sorting through drawers and wardrobes can be housekeeping as well as entertainment. Talk about the items. Talk about how they fit, how old they are, where you bought them, whether you should throw them out.

Alternatively, make a portable rummage bag for your charge to look through, with seashells, jewellery, old stamps, small balls of wool, mittens, socks, tea towels, small (unbreakable) household items, army medals, unusual buttons, a hairbrush to use or fiddle with; or woollen, cotton or furnishing scraps to finger and identify. Use anything from the past that they can find, fold, turn over, put into pairs and look at. Handling these may evoke more memories than photos can.

Pain or pleasure?

Memories that such activities evoke may be painful as well as pleasant, provoking strong emotions. Accept these and empathise, putting an arm around their shoulders or stroking their hair, hands or face if appropriate. Dementia damages the brain, but not the parts where emotions reign.

> One daughter, knowing her mother had visited many countries, brought travel books to the hospital for her to look through. She was devastated when her mother looked at the books, burst into tears and said, 'It's too hard!'

The tears were not necessarily the daughter's fault: she was doing her best. Perhaps the response shows remaining brain power, understanding and memory that the daughter assumed had gone, or perhaps books were too big an intellectual challenge. It is also quite possible that the mother would enjoy the travel books later.

If something like this happens to you, acknowledge your charge's response, and think about what prompted it.

Outings

Outings can range from visiting family and friends or going to small, quiet cafés with one or two good friends, to attending church groups or service clubs (preferably where only one person speaks most of the time), even outdoor concerts. Beside each suggestion, you may like to pencil in the names of people who could help.

Be in the audience at television cooking or other shows. A boat cruise may be fun, but for no longer than two or three hours, and try to have some form of entertainment on board, such as games, dancing or music.

Light folding chairs are sold cheaply at many supermarkets and warehouses. Some have a pocket in the arm for your drink. Use these to picnic in your garden or elsewhere: keep them in the back of your car so you can stop driving when you see something interesting, then sit and watch for a while.

You could arrange a gentle amble on a horse, through a therapeutic riding or 'riding for the disabled' programme. Take your charge to a sportsground or other open area, perhaps with your dog or grandchild (or a borrowed dog or grandchild). Take an old racket or bat to hit a ball, or collect sticks to throw, for the dog or a grandchild to retrieve, or take a golf club for your charge to swing.

At the beach, you might look under rocks for crabs or check the high-tide line to see what the sea has brought. In some parks you will find lambs, spring bulbs, birds to feed, babies, people playing sport, or brass bands: all of these are entertainment. Where there is a bridge over water, you could play Pooh Sticks; each throws a stick in one side, then go to the other side and see whose stick floats out first.

For someone whose dementia is quite advanced, arrange to sit in at a kindergarten, play centre, children's gym class, or visit a children's playground. Yes, sit on the swing, but avoid the merry-go-round and slides.

Guidelines for outings

Phone event organisers in advance to check availability of toilets, wheelchairs, seating and disability parking. Consider a trial run, to identify possible problems or challenges.

Chapter 17

Get ready early. It will take you twice as long as you expect, by the time your charge has had that snack they suddenly want, decided which jacket they'll wear, wet their pants and been changed.

Travel with fresh fruit, a drink, a cup and medications. Keep sunblock and a hat handy; sunglasses too, if your charge has them; even an umbrella as a sunshield, especially if medications make your charge sun-sensitive. Take your knitting!

Two hours (at most) outdoors can give you both the fresh air and vitamin D you need. The person you are caring for may not know if they're hot or cold, so take off or put on clothing as needed.

On the day of an event, arrive early to avoid dense crowds. Sit at the end of a row for toilet needs or early exit. Keep away from the front, remembering that the volume from some rock bands or orchestras can overwhelm. Coming home at half-time may be a good option, and keep to routine for the rest of the day. Your charge may need a longer rest than usual.

Ensure that you have options in case things don't go according to plan, and try to take everything in your stride. If all else fails, complete strangers may be willing to help.

A husband took his wife with Alzheimer's to his Toastmasters' party by taxi. They sat at the president's table, but the wife was not happy and let everyone know it. 'Who are all these people?' she said loudly. 'I don't know any of them. I want to go home.'

She persisted so he phoned for a taxi, but she continued to agitate while they waited. He, embarrassed, decided they could walk home: it was only 300 metres. His wife stopped after only a few steps, sat down on a nearby wall and wouldn't budge. He finally flagged down the only car passing – going the wrong way – whose driver kindly gave them a lift.

◆

Gloria took Doug to the beach and left him in the car while she went to get ice creams, but he collapsed into the gutter as he got out of the car on her return. Strangers helped lift him up, wipe him down and get him back into the car.

Social gatherings

Give yourself permission to scale down. If you have previously invited 15 to 30 people to fabulous meals, ask five (at the most) and plan a much less ambitious menu; for instance, drinks and nibbles rather than dinner.

Invite one of your charge's old friends (who might be living on their own) to come along. They will have lots of memories to share while you and others have more up-to-date conversation.

Sometimes invite another carer or two, with the person they are looking after. Mornings are better, as you and they tend to have more energy then than later in the day.

Celebrating festivals

If you are arranging a family meal at your home for Christmas, Diwali, Thanksgiving or another festival, you may wonder how visiting family members will react to their relative's deterioration. Let them know your situation by writing a letter or email along these lines:

> Dear ____,
>
> So glad you can join us for the family get-together after this long gap. Just in case you haven't heard our news, I'm letting you know that [X] has been diagnosed with dementia and has gone downhill since we last met.
>
> I enclose a recent photo – you'd hardly know it was the same person. Just a hint: keep questions to a minimum. Just chat about your doings, and please don't be offended if [X] doesn't seem to know who you are.
>
> [X] just needs to be treated as you would any other person. Your pleasure in seeing him, and a gentle touch on the shoulder, would mean more than you know.
>
> Would you mind phoning us just before you arrive? I'll make sure we're both ready. [X] really appreciates you coming to visit, and so do I.

Some people will not want to spend family festivities with a person with dementia. Accept this. It may be a bit hurtful but it's not a bad thing, because it keeps numbers down.

Plan for non-alcoholic drinks, and a bright entertainment area that is easily cleaned. Arrange to sing old songs and re-tell family stories; perhaps rent a seasonal video; talk about the familiar or new decorations.

You could arrange a pot-luck meal to which all contribute – a lunch or even brunch (this may help with your charge's possible sundowning collapse) – or someone else could have the get-together at their home.

Gifts for your charge

Birthday, Christmas and other gifts may be delightedly received, but can rather confuse your charge. They may be overwhelming, and better put away and doled out later, one by one. Suitable presents from you, friends and family could include the following:

- Foodstuffs – fruit-mince tarts, individual Christmas puddings, packets of sweets, fruit or biscuits.
- Music and pictures – a CD of favourite (sing-along) and soothing music of their era, a portable music player, a photo album with captions naming familiar people and places, a neighbourhood picture book showing your house and others nearby, a short comedy DVD; a waterproof radio.
- Clothing and accessories – an identity bracelet (including blood group), clothing and other items with Velcro fasteners.
- Health and well-being gifts – tokens for the podiatrist or hairdresser, a massage voucher, a shower/bath chair, a hand-held shower-head, a safe and convenient night-light, a long-handled back brush, non-stinging shampoo, bath salts or oils, an oil burner and relaxing essential oils, an orthopaedic cushion.
- Recreational/decorative gifts – a plant container, goldfish in a bowl, a soft rubber ball to squeeze in hands, larger soft balls to toss about (for instance, boccia indoor bowls), a simple jigsaw.
- Special 'quality time' – hugs and physical tenderness; a seasonal visit or trip out – even around the block; time together on 'crafts' (making cards, little boxes, simple toys, balsa wood aeroplanes with coloured paper, glue, wood, foil, cellophane, safety scissors, sandpaper, and so on).

Where to from here

- Chapter 8: Adapting the Home Environment
- Chapter 10: Wider Support and Self-care, especially 'From a distance'
- Chapter 11: Independence and Safety
- Chapter 16: Exercise
- Chapter 18: Holidays and Travel

Chapter 18

Holidays and Travel

Will we manage?

Even if you and your charge have lived and holidayed together for many years, you may be surprised at how and when dementia affects their ability to travel and stay away from home. Some carers overestimate the abilities of the person they are looking after.

> Janine's support group had their doubts about her planned visit to England with Jeffrey, and afterwards she confessed it was unwise. He had been completely disoriented on the flight, and it had been a nightmare. Once they arrived, their son and his family helped her look after him, but they were appalled by his condition and thought she'd made the wrong decision to travel.

Even then, there was a bright side – the overseas family now had a better understanding of what she was coping with.

Other people manage the challenges much better than their carers could have imagined.

> One woman, very forgetful and frail, was so scared that she wouldn't even visit her own letter-box. Despite this, two daughters took her to Sydney – a birthday trip they had planned before her illness made itself so evident.
>
> Their mother had a blissful time and went everywhere with them until, feeling extra tired one afternoon, she said to them, 'You two go on, I'll go back to the hotel.' They didn't take the chance; but wondered afterwards whether she would have found her way there.

The 'recovery' was only temporary, but still worthwhile.

This was an example of how stimulation can slow down the progress of dementia. Rallying like this can have its down side, if your charge puts on such a good show that onlookers won't believe there's a problem.

> Anthony brightened up so much when visiting his family in another city that they didn't accept he was deteriorating much at all.

A trial trip

If the person you are looking after is keen to travel overseas and you think they are up to it, do a short trial trip to visit family or friends not far away, using the form of transport you would envisage for the longer trip.

You may have passed the 'travel by' date if your charge:

- becomes disoriented or agitated fairly regularly in what should be familiar surroundings
- has continence problems
- says 'Time to go home' when out on short local visits
- is anxious, tearful or withdrawn in crowded, noisy settings
- wanders unexpectedly or seems agitated for no reason
- shows paranoia or aggressive, uninhibited behaviour or suffers from delusions.

If they are in the earlier stages of dementia and do not have these problems, you can consider travelling with them, at least in your own country. It may not be without problems, but is possible with careful planning.

Think first about your reasons for wanting to go: are they compelling? Perhaps you simply need a break. That and your budget – as well as the abilities of the person you are looking after – will influence how, where and when you go.

Holidays
A holiday at home

This is the cheapest option and the easiest, as everything is at hand: medications, incontinence equipment, special eating implements and other household aids. It is important that you avoid the usual daily grind as much as possible.

For instance, decide to do no cooking, baking, gardening, odd jobs, or anything you don't want to do. Have a rest and ignore as many routine chores as possible (you'll probably have to do some washing). Arrange for more frequent daily help with showering, dressing, and so on.

If you went away you would have to pay for your meals. So buy them: items such as tinned fruit, cereal, toast for breakfast; comfort foods or delicatessen delicacies for lunch; frozen or ready-made dinners – or go out for meals. Spend money on favourite snacks.

Amuse yourselves from the suggestions in Chapter 17: Entertainment, or your imagination. Be a tourist in your own town.

Motel or bed and breakfast

Staying at a motel or bed and breakfast in your home town is the second cheapest option, and travel to another town (or towns) to stay in such accommodation is the third cheapest. Wherever you go, consider taking a helper with you: a spare bed is often included in the tariff.

You can consult a directory for accommodation that has been inspected and graded for standard and price. Book an attractive, suitable place involving minimal travel time. Don't decide to fly, as this can be complicated by getting to and from the airport, and having to wait for flights and luggage. Consult the proprietor in advance about how they and you can meet your charge's special needs.

If you wish to move from place to place, arrange only short trips. It is less confusing, however, for a person with dementia to have to adapt to only one strange place.

Hotel

This more expensive choice offers lovely luxury! You don't even have to make your beds, and most hotels have a laundry service (though that is extra expense, and you may want to do your own washing).

Hotel accommodation is more complicated, however, with various entrances and exits to watch, and you need constant vigilance if the person you are travelling with is a wanderer.

Let the hotel know if you need a wheelchair.

Travelling to other towns

However you travel, make sure your charge is not too hot or cold. Try to have a pillow handy so they can doze comfortably en route. Know where clean toilet facilities are on the way, and have a change of clothing and medications (plus cup and water to take them with) readily available. Help your travelling companion when they get up or out: they will be stiff and may stumble.

Tips for travel by car

- Have a slightly more than basic first aid kit.
- Arrange to stop at an eating place with a good reputation. Warn the management about copious crumbs, and the reason.
- A hired car should have window-lock features – automatic windows can be dangerous for fiddling fingers.
- If possible, be a passenger, and seat the person with dementia next to the driver. You can then keep an eye on your charge from the back seat.

Comfort and mobility in cars

These suggestions apply whether the trip is short or long. In your own car, to make it easier for disabled people to position themselves, you could try the following:

- Tuck a large, thick plastic bag or sheet of plastic around the seat.
- Use a seat cover or cushion of smooth fabric or imitation leather.
- Buy a swivelling seat from a mail-order firm or hardware store.

If there is no handle above your charge's door for them to hang on to while they get in and comfortable, buy a bow-shaped handle (or two) at a hardware or auto accessories store and screw them on to the car interior roof above the passenger's window. (Avoid attaching a handle to the door frame, as this may tear the rubber seal.)

When your charge is half in or on the seat, move them the rest of the way with a gentle but firm sideways push with your hip. Know how to collapse a walker easily. Often they will not fit in the boot and are best standing folded up in the back behind a front seat.

Travel by train or bus

Long-distance trains or buses may not have disability access ramps, so you may need another helper to get your person with dementia on board, as staff may be too busy; but ask them during the trip for help in disembarking.

If you need a wheelchair for your companion during train travels, the company may prefer that it be stowed in the luggage compartment, although smaller wheelchairs may fit on board. Plan for your needs with the staff.

Ask the company what stops there will be where your charge can walk about.

Flying overseas

This is only for people with mild dementia, and if the person you are caring for has never flown, it would probably be better not to try flying. If you are confident you can manage a trip to another country:

- limit each part of the trip to somewhere two or, at the most, three hours' flight away
- go with an organised tour if possible; having a leader in charge reduces stress and uncertainty.

Arranging overseas travel

Talk to your medical specialist well in advance. Arrange medications for the whole trip and all emergencies. Include duplicate copies of your prescriptions in case you lose your baggage or medications, and carry a doctor's letter with details about your health needs. In your hand luggage, carry sufficient medications for several days and a copy of your prescriptions, in case your main luggage is lost. Check that any extra medications prescribed for the trip, such as for altitude sickness, are compatible with your present ones. Work out with your doctor, specialist or support organisation how to manage medications and meals in relation to time-zone changes.

Let the travel agent know your companion's level of disability, including their memory loss. Avoid fast-moving sight-seeing trips; but escorted tours, with a group of people you know and who understand your situation, may be enjoyable.

Allow time for a stopover, arranging longer than usual stopovers if there are time differences for your charge to adjust to. Many major airports have shower, massage and nap facilities such as a stopover bed in the transit lounge. Before your trip, find out online (or ask your travel agent) about these and print off a map showing their locations. Ask in advance for a bed to be made available.

Ask the agent to locate suitable accommodation. Let them or the tour operator know about medications you will carry.

Make sure both of you are eligible for insurance, search around for the best terms, and let the insurer know about pre-existing medical conditions. For an extra charge you can usually receive full cover.

Be ready for unexpected diversions or having to cancel the trip. Ask your travel agent to find a holiday package that allows you to leave the tour early without financial penalty – or consider insurance for this too – in case your companion becomes ill or restive.

Airline staff will provide food for almost any dietary needs, and at any time required, but do book your special meals in advance. Ask for an aisle seat, preferably at the rear near the toilets.

Inform the airline, hotels and tour operators about your companion's special needs (wheelchairs, meals and so on), their memory loss and if they should not be left on their own. The airline may require you to fill out a form about these matters in advance, and have your doctor sign it. Most airlines will, if forewarned, provide oxygen for anyone with dementia if the lack of oxygen in the plane produces hallucinations.

You can also arrange for a wheelchair at the airport. This can come with a meet-and-assist service which helps clients through airport ticketing and customs (blissful).

What to tell your travel companion

Prepare your charge for the trip in a manner relevant to the extent of their dementia. What and when you tell them depends on their potential to worry about the plans or to forget – repeatedly.

Julia's mother seemed excited at the prospect of spending a week with her brother in Auckland. Julia took her to buy the plane tickets, came home and said, 'Well, wasn't it good getting the tickets?'
'What tickets?'
'For Auckland...'
'Where?'
'You know, at Air New Zealand.'
'No, what were they for?'
'Auckland.' And so on...

You can tell them well in advance and ask them to help you prepare. Or you can give short notice: 'We're going to Sydney tomorrow. I'm going to start packing some of your things. Would you like to help me?' Or you can just announce your plans not long before you leave.

Other preparations

Be prepared to do everything for the two of you.

Leave details of your travel schedule with family members back home. Put duplicate copies of important documents in special safe places.

Have an identification bracelet for your charge to wear. In their pocket, put your name along with the address and phone number of your next destination. You will need to change this if (or as) you move around.

If you plan to take a mobile phone, you would be wise to check costs and availability of the 'roaming' mode where you are going. To avoid unnecessary expense, program your phone to divert all calls to voicemail, then use text messaging to communicate.

Invest in (or borrow) lightweight, wheeled luggage, including perhaps a shoulder bag you can sling diagonally (this is easier for you to get at and may be more secure than a backpack). Pack a minimal amount. Make sure all your clothing for the trip is named, comfortable and is made from easy-care fabric for washing. Have a change of clothing in your carry-on bag.

Ideally you should be rested when you set out. Checking your luggage through to a final destination will remove some of the stress of travelling, too. Be ready to be seated before other passengers (ask to board early, with others who need help) and wait to be last off.

While travelling

If you have a companion of the opposite sex, contact a crew member early and explain that you will need someone to help them use the toilet. To cover emergencies, a continence pad may be a good idea (although these are difficult to manage in a confined space).

Security regulations mean you can't carry water for medications on to an international flight, but you can usually fill an empty bottle on the plane or in airport toilets.

Carry a hat or cap to shield your charge from the heat, and avoid sitting on the sunny side of buses or trains. Help your companion with their seatbelt, open their window or adjust their window curtains or sunshade.

You will probably have researched a few local sights beforehand, but on arrival get local tourist pamphlets to find out more. Choose eating places and restaurants where crumbs under the table and dropped food are not of too much concern.

Things to avoid

- ✦ Avoid putting all medications and prescriptions in one place in case that bag is lost. Keep some with you at all times, and split the rest between bags.
- ✦ Stay away from busy places such as city streets or large amusement parks. They may cause your charge to become overstimulated or anxious. Visiting a relative with a large family can be confusing for your charge too.
- ✦ Avoid buying heavy or awkward keepsakes or gifts. If you must, mail them home.
- ✦ Avoid asking a stranger to look after your charge, even for a short spell. A person who doesn't understand dementia won't know how to react in a difficult situation.

Exercises for both of you on a plane

Sit well back into your seat. In the small of your back use a lumbar roll, or a fat, soft, rolled-up towel held with stout rubber bands.

Keep ankles moving: pump your feet up and down and circle them both ways; march on the spot in your seats, lifting alternate knees up and down. Straighten legs – out in front and then down (space permitting). Reach arms out in front and above your head (space permitting).

Change the weight on your bottom by rocking from side to side and by pushing up with your hands on your arm-rests. Walk the aisles frequently; stand in the space by the toilets doing deep breathing, going up and down on your toes and stretching for minutes.

Ten time tips

1. Time your travel to coincide with your companion's best daily periods.
2. Arrange only one activity a day, with a couple of alternatives up your sleeve.
3. Include breaks along the way for rest, snacks, medications, fluids, toilet stops.
4. Plan places to rest each day.
5. Leave more time for transfers between trains or planes, or spend an extra night or two in one place to allow for more leisurely sightseeing.
6. Anticipate and avoid delays. If you are travelling by bus, have a friend drive you to the departure point; or take a taxi, so you don't have to handle the luggage. If going by train or plane, go by taxi or shuttle bus for the same reason and door-to-door service.
7. Always call ahead to make sure the transport is leaving on time.
8. In case you are unavoidably delayed, always carry medications, some water to take them with, and something to pass the time, such as cards, crosswords, puzzles, Walkman, iPod loaded with favourite tunes and programmes, iPhone.
9. An hour-by-hour itinerary will help you to identify, and prepare for, the pressure points.
10. Allow extra time for everything.

Familiarity and strangeness

The strange new surroundings of your accommodation may worry your companion. Leave bathroom lights on all night. Have the first shower yourself and check the water temperature. Turn on your charge's shower, as unfamiliar knobs can be confusing to a person with dementia.

Make sure the unit/bedroom doors are locked to prevent your companion from wandering in the strange place. You could activate the door safety-catch at nights and place a chair in front of the door, having made plans should there be a fire.

Note all fire exits and their position in relation to your room. This is not only in case of fire: your charge may go for a walk down the fire stairs.

While you are away, keep to daily routines, with baths or showers at the same time as at home. But your charge may enjoy a spa pool instead of a bath.

Maintain familiar eating habits. Go to places where there are the same types of food your charge has at home. Don't go to crowded restaurants with exotic menus if they are used to eating quietly at home. Use room service, or choose a restaurant table where you can eat in a quiet corner.

Have confidence in your special knowledge about the person you are caring for. You know what works and what doesn't, and they do too.

Make the most of what comes, accept the ups and downs as cheerfully as you can, and laugh a lot with them about the funny things that happen along the way. Relax and enjoy your holiday together.

> Ann and Reg were offered a free stay in a Fijian resort. Reg had moderate dementia, and they asked for and were given the 'disability suite'. It had handles by the bath and toilet, a toilet overseat, and was near the informal lunch bar and swimming pool. There Reg dog-paddled a bit, but mainly walked up and down in the waist-high water – very good exercise. The two spent every day lazing on deck chairs with a regular supply of cool drinks from friendly waiters; and every night had a choice of dining places.
>
> One afternoon, as they walked very slowly along the grass beach frontage, Ann missed her sunglasses. She sat Reg down on a seat under a shady palm tree, asked him to wait and dashed off to get them. Five minutes later she returned: no sign of him.
>
> Ann quickly walked in one direction as far as he could have gone. No! She returned and went in the other direction. Not there!

She ran to the main lobby and then to their room. No. Alarmed, she returned to the seat. He wouldn't have walked into the sea? Just then, a waiter came across to her.

'Are you looking for your hubby, ma'am?' he enquired, smiling broadly.

'Yes! Have you seen him?'

'Yes, ma'am. I found him walking along the grass looking lost and I thought he should be rescued, so I took him and he's in a deck chair by the pool. He's a nice gentleman.'

Ann joined Reg at the pool. She never mentioned her worry to him, but that was the last time she let him out of her sight in Fiji.

Where to from here

- Chapter 9: Managing Difficult Behaviour
- Chapter 11: Independence and Safety
- Chapter 12: Feelings
- Chapter 17: Entertainment, especially 'Outings'
- Chapter 19: Eating and Drinking
- Chapter 21: Toileting, especially 'Toileting tips'
- Chapter 22: Wandering

PART FIVE

Practical Strategies for Managing

Chapter 19

Eating and Drinking

Although dementia affects each person differently, most will probably still enjoy their food; so keep meals interesting and tasty – for your benefit as well as theirs – and surroundings as normal as possible. Each person will deteriorate in their own way, with changes leading sometimes to messy eating or even refusal at times to eat or drink, and slow eaters taking 30 or 40 minutes to complete their meal.

When Helen went away, Bruce and Alison asked Donald to have lunch with them one day. The difference between the two men was amazing.

Donald, an 18-year veteran of Parkinson's and dementia, had involuntary movements from long-term medication use – but he handled his knife and fork with delicacy and ate very tidily. Bruce had had Lewy body dementia for only five years; he was a social disaster, pushing food out of his high-sided plate and having to use his fingers, but he was unembarrassed and wore his bib without complaint.

He and Donald talked in their quiet voices with obvious good fellowship, in spurts of chat and silence. Donald said he'd been given a disability bib at day care, and had told Helen that he'd start a new business manufacturing them: 'It's a growth market!' he'd commented.

When messy eating is a problem

Eat in the kitchen mostly, or at an outside table if it is warm and sunny, but have the main meal of the day at its regular place.

When balance and muscles deteriorate, it can be useful for your charge to have a chair that gives support during meals. A sturdy but light orthopaedic chair with arms, supportive back and soft, comfortable, washable seat can be obtained from your visiting occupational therapist. The arms enable the person you are looking after to pull their chair up to the table. If they can't manage that, move the table to them; or stand them facing and against the table, bring up the chair yourself and push it under their knees to let them sit down easily.

Accessories and implements

Guard the carpet under their chair with at least two metres of metre-wide clear, heavy-duty plastic sheeting with a 'pronged' finish on the back. If the floor is polished or vinyl, of course, you don't need the plastic; you can mop the floor clean.

> David, who had Lewy body dementia, didn't think he had any problems at mealtimes, but he drove his wife crazy as the fingers of his left hand (he ate with a spoon in his right hand) gradually crept on to his plate and finished up crawling round in the middle of his food. 'Watch your left hand, Dave,' she would say, and he would look at it and move it to the side, but then it would start crawling again. It ended up needing a good wash afterwards, as did the table and floor around him.

If the napkin you tuck in their collar isn't sufficient, put on an easily-washed smock, or button-up shirt (put on back-to-front) or apron (tied round the neck) to protect clothing from spilled food and drink. Tuck the edge of the smock, shirt or other garment under the plate in front of them. This will catch most dropped food.

Otherwise you could buy four large, practical bibs at a disability centre, or make them yourself. They should be:
- made of good-quality, durable, non-absorbent polyester material with waterproof backing, easily washed and simple to put on
- fastened round the neck with a dome, or tied with tapes
- shoulder-width and reaching to below the waist, turned up at the bottom front to form a pocket to catch dropped food.

Have a good supply of easily laundered or 'wipe over' table cloths or mats. Avoid patterned ones: the person with dementia may spend time trying to pick up and eat the different small 'bits' they see.

Serve each course in a glass or earthenware pie plate, placed on a damp cloth or tea towel. This, plus its weight, stops it from being pushed around too much, and the vertical sides of the plate prevent food falling off the edge. The sides are also easy to push food against, to heap it on to spoon or fork. (Disability centres have plates of different sizes and shapes, made especially for people with eating problems.) Take a special high-sided plate – and bib – when you go out for meals.

> Alan and Judy were invited to have dinner at Lynne and Alastair's home. Judy offered to bring Alan's special plate, but 'No,' said Lynne, 'we don't want any fuss; he can't do any damage.'
>
> Afterwards, as Judy collected a cupful of Alan's dinner off the table where he'd been, and then swept up copious amounts of rice, chicken and vegetables from the floor and rug under Alan's chair, she berated herself. The neighbours had had no idea of what they were letting themselves in for.

Your charge may prefer to use their familiar cutlery, but all sorts are available at disability centres; take them there to choose for themselves. As disability increases, spoons are easier to manage than knives or forks.

When it comes to drinks, use a transparent cup to see where the liquid level is when you are helping the person to drink: tinted glass mugs are good. Don't put very hot liquids in a plastic mug as it may crack. Bendable straws from supermarkets are useful in glasses or mugs if they can manage them.

Try a child's training cup when they can't hold other drinking vessels. It has two handles and a spill-proof cover with a spout. Similar, less childish-looking porcelain mugs are available at disability centres.

Food and drink
A balanced diet

Try to offer at least five servings of fruit and vegetables each day. 'Filler-ups' could be breads and cereals, pasta, rice and other grain products – wholegrain varieties preferred – several times a day if possible. Have at least two servings of low-fat milk or milk products (yoghurt or cheese) daily, as well as lean meats and poultry, with fish on the menu at least once a week.

Be relaxed about allowing fads. If ice cream is all they want, give it to them, but ask your doctor or dietician about the possible need for supplements.

Size and texture

Cut everything into bite-sized portions if necessary. Be prepared to change to 'finger foods' when coordination with cutlery fails, such as sandwiches, chicken drumsticks, pieces of fruit and other soft, thick edibles (make sure that tricky bones and pips are removed). Cut peeled fruit into bite-sized pieces, or pull oranges or mandarins into segments. Serve these as finger food or with a small dessert fork in a high-sided plate.

When they need softer foods:
- offer minced chicken and vegetables, mashed potatoes, scrambled eggs or soft omelettes, well-mashed fish in tasty sauce
- try jellies made with nutritious fruit juices, stewed apples and other fruit which can produce a purée, ice creams, frozen yoghurt, porridge in gruel form, milk-softened cereal 'biscuits', and so on
- continue to offer a fibre-rich diet with fruit, vegetables, wholemeal bread and cereals containing wheat, bran or oats – all mashed as much as necessary.

Tips for eating and drinking

- Eat the main meal in the middle of the day.
- Offer more small snacks during the day, if your charge gets tired during mealtimes.
- Avoid talking during meals.
- Sit upright when eating.
- Take small bites and chew well before swallowing; pause between mouthfuls.
- Swallow food before taking a sip of fluid, rather than washing down food with drink.
- Identify and avoid foods that are difficult to handle, eat or digest.

Getting enough fluids

Include a drink or other liquid in most meals, since medications may reduce saliva. Offer gravy, sauces, a glass of water or fruit juice.

Regular drinks are important: make sure your charge has them. Eight cups of liquids replace the fluids we lose each day, lubricate the body and help prevent constipation. Jellies, ice-blocks and ice cream count as liquids. Go easy, though, on drinks containing caffeine or alcohol (see 'Alcoholic drinks' below).

Low fluid intake can bring dehydration with symptoms such as flushing, fever, rapid pulse, dizziness, confusion, and vomiting. (See also Chapter 15: Maintaining Health 'Checking for dehydration'.) It can also lead to urinary tract infections.

Help with swallowing

In the later stages of several dementias, people may have difficulty chewing or swallowing, or may tend to choke. 'Thin' liquids such as water, tea or coffee can make them cough. If your charge has these problems, liquidise solids to a thick, soup-like consistency. To prevent choking, thicken most liquids to the same consistency (your pharmacist may have commercial thickeners). Tomato juice is a good, naturally thick drink, as is milk.

When they are taking a drink, encourage small sips and slow drinking. Be extra careful when they're nearly finished. Have them leave the last drops, and not tip their head back to get the liquid down, as this can lead to choking. Instead, suggest they tuck their chin in slightly and keep the mouthful until they are ready to swallow. Pay particular attention, too, if they are using a straw.

Make sure a cold drink really is cold, and put something a bit sour – lime or lemon – into water. Sucking on a small chip of ice can help swallowing, and fizzy drinks can be easier for some. Reheat a hot drink when your charge is halfway through, if necessary.

Keep in touch with your doctor over swallowing problems, and perhaps consult a speech therapist. A Parkinson's patient whose muscles slow down may be able to adapt their eating, but people in the last stages of Alzheimer's actually forget how to swallow.

Warning signs

Be extra-alert with food and drink if your charge develops any of the following:
- obvious difficulty in chewing/swallowing/controlling food or drink in their mouth
- dribbling food or drink from their mouth
- food apparently sticking in their mouth or throat, or food left in their mouth after swallowing
- coughing or clearing their throat, or gurgling/wet-sounding voice, during or immediately after eating or drinking
- taking longer to eat meals; reluctance to eat or drink, unexplained weight loss
- chestiness or repeated chest infections.

If you notice such changes, tell your doctor.

Choking emergencies – the Heimlich manoeuvre

If the person you are looking after chokes, can't catch their breath and turns red and then purple:
1. Quickly stand close behind them.
2. Put your arms under their armpits.
3. Join your hands in front over their stomach and just under their ribs.
4. Brace yourself against them.
5. Give a short, violent backwards tug.

This should cause them to projectile-vomit immediately, bringing up whatever was sticking in their throat and allowing them to breathe again.

Too little ... or too much
Encourage a reluctant eater

Sometimes, after you have seated your charge at the table, they go on strike. Avoid arguing. Instead, put on some quiet, favourite music, and massage their shoulders and neck while standing chatting behind them, to relax them and show your empathy. (Ensure first that they are in the mood to be touched.)

Moisten their lips with a taste of their meal, or ask them simply to savour the smell. This may get them started. If it doesn't work – and if medications permit – try an occasional small wine or sherry before a meal, to start them thinking of eating.

A snack of vegetable soup in a mug, accompanied by a slice of toast or croutons, is a good alternative way of getting calories into a person with dementia. Otherwise, snacks in drink form can be made with blended yoghurt, fresh fruit, ice cream and/or milk, or egg nogs.

There are also tasty, calorie-laden drinks in small cardboard cartons, which come in several flavours, with diabetic options as well. Your doctor may be able to write a prescription for a free permanent supply from your pharmacy. If the person with dementia continues to refuse regular meals and is losing weight, try giving them their nutrition in regular small snacks throughout the day.

People with Alzheimer's and Parkinson's dementia seem to lose weight more rapidly than those with other dementias, even with adequate nutrition, so catering for them may require particular effort.

> Loss of weight was a side-effect of Bruce's condition, so Alison always cooked meals he would enjoy. She served them on colourful, easily washed mats and gave him 'wine' (a soft drink) in a wineglass, since he longed for things to be normal.
>
> As the years passed, the wineglass was dispensed with and he became less able to control his fork (then the spoon he moved on to). Because he would not let Alison feed him, increasing piles of meat and vegetables landed up in his bib or on the floor.
>
> His wife would get up from her dinner, give him a hug and a kiss on the back of his neck, unobtrusively gathering up the bib and emptying it into his plate. Bruce scarcely noticed and would continue eating.
>
> He always wanted ice cream afterwards, but could take 15–20 minutes with the first course and be very tired by the time dessert came. While he ploughed on, Alison would move to the end of the table to work on a jigsaw, or excuse herself and do the dishes.
>
> Returning, she sometimes found Bruce asleep in his chair, his nose in the ice cream.

If you are concerned about weight loss, speak with your doctor about supplements; in particular, agitated or very active people with dementia may need them. Also ask for an appointment with a dietician. Perhaps your charge needs more exercise to stimulate their appetite?

Changes in eating habits and constant lack of appetite can indicate depression. Definitely tell your doctor if it persists.

'When are we eating?'

Sometimes people with dementia forget they have just had a meal and ask 'When are we eating?' or say they never get anything to eat. This is probably because the disease has affected the so-called 'satiety centre' in the brain. If you can't distract them with another activity, offer a non-fattening snack of raw carrot, celery or rusk.

Alcoholic drinks

Sometimes people with dementia forget that they have just had a drink and ask for, or pour themselves, another. This is good if the drink is non-alcoholic, but disastrous if it is not. Alcohol often does not mix with medications, and should therefore be unobtrusively but carefully monitored, and hidden if necessary. If they insist they want a drink, serve tonic or something else non-alcoholic in a wineglass, or non-alcoholic beer in a tumbler.

If your charge is in the habit of taking an alcoholic drink before supper, let them – as long as they don't overdo it, and it doesn't conflict with their medications. If, however, they are turning into an alcoholic in their dementia, try subtle strategies. These could include limiting spending money or, if necessary, telling liquor store staff about the dementia and asking them not to sell alcohol to your charge (show them a doctor's note, if you need to). You could also fill spirit bottles with coloured water, or water down the colourless ones.

Beatrice spent several weeks in hospital after breaking her leg. She had been over-indulging in alcohol even before she began developing Alzheimer's, so the family was delighted by this unplanned withdrawal period.

On her first night after her discharge, staying with her son, she received her pre-dinner lemon, lime and bitters – minus the usual alcoholic addition. After downing a second glass Beatrice said gaily to him, 'I'm feeling ever so nicely, dear. Just as well I don't have to drive home, isn't it?'

Eating out

Dress up for a change and ask one or two friends (at most) to join you. Choose a quiet and well-lit restaurant so your charge is less likely to feel overwhelmed.

Phone up first, request an out-of-the-way table, tell them you will be bringing someone with a disability, ask to be excused for any mess you make, and request fast service.

Hand a card to the waiter printed with 'My friend is not well. I shall order for us both. Please take answers to any questions from me.' However, let the person with dementia give their own order if they can read the menu. Otherwise read it to them and let them choose, or order for them unobtrusively.

Preserve the dignity of the person you are looking after. Having warned the management, don't take their usual bib, and consider whether to take along their special, high-sided plate. Dress them in easily laundered clothes and let them use the restaurant napkins.

Where to from here

- Chapter 8: Adapting the Home Environment
- Chapter 11: Independence and Safety
- Chapter 15: Maintaining Health, especially 'Checking for dehydration'
- Chapter 16: Exercise
- Chapter 17: Entertainment, especially 'Cooking'
- Chapter 21: Toileting
- Chapter 25: Choosing Full-time Care, 'Food'
- Chapter 26: Moving into Full-time Care, 'Weight loss'

Chapter 20

Showering and Dressing

As dementia takes over, spills and other mishaps occur, no matter how fastidious the person was previously. You may feel that the daily all-over bath, twice-daily dressing and undressing (more, given toilet accidents) dominate your life. Then there's the wiping and washing of your home. It all adds up, as time goes by.

Alison showered and dressed Bruce for months until one morning, as she was putting on Bruce's socks, pain shot through her back – an old injury had flared up. She phoned the special support person assigned to her by the hospital. Yes, someone would come in each morning to shower and dress Bruce.

He wasn't happy. 'They send a different person every day!' he complained. He didn't want these strangers being so intimate.

'I just can't do it any longer, darling,' Alison told him. 'My back is kaput again. Do you remember when you had to look after me years ago, when I spent a week flat on my back? That prolapsed disc? It's almost that bad again.'

Bruce understood and didn't complain much afterwards; but he identified his ideal helper – the beautiful Indian woman. Alison let her needs assessor know, and the empathetic aide became one of Bruce's favourite visitors as they settled into a comfortable and, for his wife, less demanding daily routine.

Some people have never been undressed in front of anyone else. Your charge may be indignant when strangers come to shower and dress them.

Introduce these helpers as tactfully as you can. They are used to relating easily to different patients, and should be sensitive to the wishes of each.

Find out what light and practicable cover your person with dementia can wear while going to be showered and, afterwards, going to be dressed. A wrap-around robe may do the trick, or at least wrap a towel around them. Their privacy and dignity need to be respected.

Showering

An outward-swinging shower door can be propped open, if necessary, for better access. Washing the far side of your charge is hard, however, and they find it hard to turn, even if grab rails have been installed and they hear and understand what you are asking. One solution, if you are their partner, is to shower with them; another is to wear all-over raingear. This may elicit shrieks of laughter or dismay. But it's worth trying.

At first the person you are caring for will be able to stand and shower themselves. Later they may be more secure sitting on a stool, and being helped. Much later you may need to get a hoist to lift them off their bed and on to a shower-wheelchair. You should have home helpers for this.

A man who looked after his wife for several years came up with a different solution:

> When Lochie decided that Stella needed a thorough wash he dressed himself (with bathing trunks instead of underpants), packed a bag with three towels, her clothes for the day and his underwear, and drove her in her dressing gown to the local heated swimming pool. Having phoned in advance, he was given the key to the pool's special unit for disabled people.
>
> This was warm enough for him to strip before he undressed Stella, turned on the warm shower and took both of them under it together. Lochie was able to wash her hair and soap her all over, more thoroughly than at home.
>
> His wife enjoyed the togetherness and the long, warm rinse afterwards. Lochie would then towel them both dry, sit Stella on another dry towel on the wooden bench and dress her, before doing the same for himself.

If your charge prefers a bath

You are best to discourage baths, as getting in and out becomes increasingly dangerous. But some people with dementia just love to wallow in warm water, so let them if possible. As when showering, help them remove clothes in the bedroom and put a wrap round them. If it is chilly, have the bathroom heated.

If the person you are caring for runs the bath themselves, check the depth and temperature before they get in. Bath oils in the water will moisturise the skin but can make the bath slippery. Tomato juice in the bath is supposed to help dispel persistent body odours.

Getting in

1. Put the stool – with a towel on top to help with comfort and turning – beside the bath.
2. Sit them on the stool facing you.
3. Say, 'Good. Can you swing your legs round over the side? The water's nice and warm. Give me your hand. I'll pour some warm water over it. Is that all right?'
4. Keep the person steady, while swinging their legs around over the side and into the bath.
5. They lean forward, use one hand to hold the handle on the opposite wall, and hold on to you with their other hand to steady themselves.
6. Semi-standing, they turn sideways to face the taps (still holding the opposite handle) and sit down.

Your charge should be able to soak safely in the bath by themselves. They may be able to wash themselves, or you may kneel by the bath to help. Don't stand and bend over: you may hurt your back.

Getting out

When they are ready to get out, do the actions in reverse, with lots of help and steadying.
1. They stand or squat in the bath holding its handles or your hand.
2. Next they turn and push their bottom over the side, onto the towel-covered stool.

3. They swing (or you pull) their legs around, over the side and down onto the bathmat.
4. Finally they stand up and dry themselves, or are dried.

If you find they cannot sit up to get out, try using an extra-large bath towel, or about 2 metres of soft material (butter muslin?). Fold this three or four times lengthwise, then put it round their upper back and under their arms as they lie in the water.

1. You hold both ends. As they try to lift themselves (using the handles on the side/s of the bath), gently pull them up to a sitting position.
2. Ease them over onto all fours and, with help, to a standing position.
3. Once they are upright, put both ends of the towel in one hand, leaving your other hand and arm free to assist and steady while they step out over the edge (still with the towel under their arms for support), or sit on the stool to get out.

Alternatives

If your charge prefers a 'bed sponge' or 'flannel wash' to a bath or shower, it is best not to argue. Some people have washed, or been washed, that way for years. Your charge may later change their mind and even bathe at day care, if that place has facilities.

Older people often did not bathe every day when they were young. Certainly, during times of war, poverty and depression, fuel and money for heating water were scarce, and two inches of warm water in the weekly bath was the ration, and sometimes others shared it. No one dies for want of a daily wash.

Reluctance to wash

People with dementia are sticklers for routine, but sometimes they will object strongly to washing. You have several choices:
- ✦ Tempt them by buying them their own special, attractive face cloth or sponge.
- ✦ Give them a 'top and tail' wash with a flannel.
- ✦ Let them wash you first.
- ✦ Leave washing until tomorrow.

Trevor would occasionally lie in bed and refuse to get up. To begin with, Connie would urge him to be ready for the helper. 'Too tired. Feeling rotten,' he'd mumble.

When the helper arrived, Connie would tell them that Trevor was feeling 'anti' this morning. 'Not to worry. Leave him to me,' the woman would say, and would saunter through to the bedroom calling out, 'Hullooo, hulloo, Trevor, it's me,' and cope in her own way.

When Trevor knew this helper well and liked her, Connie would walk round the block for some necessary exercise, even when he was 'on strike'. The woman usually sat on the bed and chatted to him for a while and he ended up having the 'blooming shower' – or sometimes he just had a sponge wash, sitting in a chair. Sometimes they understandingly left him in bed and went on to their next client when Connie returned.

If they have not bathed for two or three days and really need attention, be firm but – if they have early or moderate dementia – offer them a choice: 'Will you have an all-over-on-the-bed-wash or a bath or shower?' or 'Will you have your shower now or before you go to bed?' Otherwise be matter-of-fact: 'Your bath is ready now.'

Although it is good to let the person you are caring for make their own decisions, you can't let them avoid washing for too long: unwashed, unhygienic skin can erupt unpleasantly.

Wash-time tips

Plan to have wash-time at the same time every day.

'Bathing at night is usually best – relaxing and tiring, and just pyjamas to put on afterwards – sleep is better,' one carer reported.

Some people with dementia put in the plug, wash their hands or their shaving brush, and leave the taps running.

The first two times Bronson overflowed the basin, the insurance company paid to have the bathroom carpet dried, and said nothing. They complained the third time, and Cheryl had the floor covered in vinyl before the fourth.

Personal grooming
Cleaning teeth

An electric toothbrush is better for teeth and gums than a manual toothbrush, but introducing one for the first time may be tricky.

Encourage teeth cleaning once or twice a day – preferably morning and night – but don't fuss too much if it leads to antagonism. Caries or gum disease may be preferable to the aggression you may have to cope with if you insist.

If your charge has forgotten what to do, show them how, making up your own short, one-at-a-time instructions. Brush your own teeth at the same time, so they can imitate you. Be prepared later to clean their teeth yourself.

Caring for nails

Keep nails short to avoid scratching. Clip them after bathing, when they are softer. Use scissors or clippers, whichever is easier. Apply nail polish or not, as your charge requests: clear or colour – it's their choice. If nail care is difficult, make regular appointments with an amenable podiatrist or manicurist.

Washing and styling hair

Buy baby shampoo, as it doesn't sting the eyes. Your charge will wash their own hair for a while, but will need help eventually.

Perhaps you will wash their hair in the shower, using the shower-head on the flexible hose, or in the bath. In this case, hold a wash cloth against their hair line to keep water out of their eyes as you rinse off the shampoo using a plastic mug. Always check their scalp for skin problems.

You may, of course, wash their hair with them sitting on the bathroom stool and leaning forward over the basin, or you could invest in a basin clip-on, which allows them to sit and lean their head backwards.

Look for an understanding hairdresser if you need to use one. Confer with the person with dementia over what style they want, using hairstyling books if necessary. Let them choose whether they have shorter or longer hair.

One woman with dementia in a 'special' unit always made sure her outfits were stylish and her hair well groomed. The staff let her know about mealtimes and special events, and she would arrive looking immaculate.

After that home closed and the woman had to move to another, her niece was appalled to find her without her dentures, her hair cropped, and wearing someone else's shapeless un-ironed dress. 'Oh, I don't care what I look like,' the aunt muttered morosely. 'Nothing matters any more.' The new home was keeping her clean, dressed and fed, but it was ignoring her personality.

Shaving

Shaving for a man can become very difficult. He can leave patches of stubble all over his face, whether he's using a safety razor or an electric shaver. Nevertheless, compliment him on doing a good job. This creates a much better atmosphere than nagging, and it is great that he still wants to do it. Alternatively he can grow a beard. It may make him look very distinguished. The local hairdresser may trim senior citizens' beards for only a small charge.

Getting dressed
Routines

It is preferable to have one place where your person with dementia gets dressed for the day, and a different place where they get into their nightwear. This helps them know which time of day it is.

Encourage them to choose their clothes for the day if they wish; but, if they dither, give them just two outfits to choose from. If they insist on wearing the same clothing every day, and cause a rumpus when it is in the wash, buy identical outfits. Put away other seasons' inappropriate clothing.

Put out any ointments with the clothes, so that you (or the daily helper) remember to apply them before dressing your charge.

While they are undressed, check skin for rashes or sores. See your doctor immediately if any red areas, spots or sores appear. Pressure sores or ulcers can form quickly on people who are sitting or lying much of the time, and rashes are not uncommon side-effects of medications.

Take time to apply moisturisers and make-up, if used. Moisturisers may be available on prescription.

As with other activities in this chapter, independence is ideal, but over time you will need to take over.

> Cheryl let Bronson shower and dress himself for as long as possible. She would sit and chat to him after his shower, making little comment when he came into the bedroom still glistening with water. She would pat him dry before he put his clothes on.
>
> She worried as he stood unsteadily on one leg, then the other, to put on his underpants and trousers – but she didn't say anything. Bronson's balance was pretty good for many months; but finally he could no longer balance on one leg, and had to wedge himself into a corner to get into his underpants.
>
> Cheryl gradually and unobtrusively did more and more to help him.

Too many or not enough?

If your charge puts on several layers of odd clothing, don't make too much of a fuss. You may be embarrassed, but they won't be! The clothes can be removed if they become uncomfortably hot.

If they start undressing in public, thwart them by using clothes that fasten down the back. Do, however, ask yourself why they are undressing: they could be too hot, or bored. They may be tired and wanting to get into bed; or they may simply need to go to the bathroom.

When your charge cannot dress themselves

Dry them after their shower, drape them modestly in a dry towel and take them through to the bedroom, warmed by a heater, where clothes are ready. Leave the towel around their shoulders to keep them warm while they are dressing.

Invent your own small steps in the dressing routine: as the person becomes more impaired, you may need to break the routine into even smaller steps. It can be an extremely slow business; but becomes one of your satisfying achievements for the day.

Take care you don't strain the arms or legs of either of you as you move limbs to put garments on. As the disease progresses, muscles weaken and begin to break down. This makes dressing difficult, especially for the helper.

>Doug's arms stiffened and were not easy to get clothes on, especially since he reversed instructions. 'Right arm up, please Doug,' Gloria would say, and his bent left arm would go forward!

If your charge resists getting changed for bed, you could either do it at a different time, or give it a miss. We don't have to wear nightgowns or pyjamas to bed – we can sleep in clothes, and lots of ordinary people choose to sleep naked. On cold nights it's a good idea to put your charge in a bed jacket, or even a track suit, if bed clothes may slip off.

Clothing for men and women
To choose or buy

Build up a collection of clothes that are easy to put on. Plain materials or very simple patterns are best, with no more than two coordinating colours that your charge likes. Maintaining individuality and personal dignity is important – and remember that everyone likes to dress up and look their best at formal occasions.

All clothing should be easy to wash, and need little or no ironing. When your person with dementia starts going in for respite care, items must be strong enough to withstand both washing and drying machines. Such facilities will issue a clothing list.

Buy new garments one size larger, for ease of putting on and comfort, and in case they shrink. Choose T-shirts which look okay even if they have been put on backwards.

For women who have trouble putting on a bra, try using a close-fitting cotton vest or spencer, or a maternity bra fastening in front.

For men, you will find it useful to have three or four cotton nightshirts or pairs of cotton pyjamas (with short or long legs), perhaps fleecy-lined ones for winter. All trousers should have elastic waists, and a few spare pairs of cotton pyjama pants are good to have for incontinence emergencies. Nightshirts and short pyjamas are particularly useful for easy toilet access. For women, choose short nighties (cool or warm, for the season).

Your charge's wardrobe should include three warm all-weather jackets, preferably with open-zip-up fronts or Velcro fasteners rather than buttons or toggles (this advice about fasteners applies to most clothing). Make sure the zips are good quality and don't pull open.

Two or three light summer cardigans will make a change from jackets. Remember, though, that older people may prefer warm cardigans, as they can feel cold even in the heat of summer.

Keep several identical pairs of socks for men, or knee-high stockings for women, so that you always have a match. Long, sporting socks are warmer and easier to put on than others.

Two or three pairs of woollen mittens or gloves may be a sensible purchase for someone who has icy-cold hands. Additionally, pocket hand-warmers are available at most sports apparel shops. After being immersed in boiling water for five minutes they will keep hands warm for up to 90 minutes when held in pockets. (Check that they are not too hot before use.)

A long-handled shoehorn is useful for levering shoes. All footwear should have low, flat heels. For everyday wear, choose two or three pairs of either:

- moccasins
- shoes that close with Velcro
- sneakers, or
- solid leather sandals fastened with Velcro.

The sandals can be worn with or without socks in winter and summer. Add one pair of more fashionable women's shoes, or shiny black moccasin-style slip-on men's shoes, for best wear. Stretchy laces can make lace-up shoes fairly easy to slip on and off.

Have fleecy-lined, light, zip-up boots for winter. Slippers should fit well and have non-skid soles.

If your charge is incontinent, buy two or three pairs of light, rubber-soled canvas shoes which can go through the washing machine cycle without being damaged.

To alter or make

Blouses, shirts, pyjamas and so on can be cut and hemmed down the centre back and fastened at the top with Velcro. They will look 'normal' from the front but changing will be easier. Consider having open-ended zips down the back of dresses and nightgowns. This makes dressing easier if your female charge grasps clothes tightly or struggles as you dress them.

Elsewhere, you could replace buttons, hooks, zips and belt buckles with Velcro fasteners, but only if it will not irritate skin.

For good warmth, make a wrap-around, floor-length skirt out of a cuddle rug. Fasten it with Velcro at the waist, and put it on over frocks or skirts in cold weather.

To protect fragile skin on legs, place one layer of bubble-wrap plastic between two layers of lightweight material shaped to the legs, sew it up on a sewing machine and secure with Velcro. This may need careful washing, however.

Once your charge is bedridden, instead of a hospital gown, split loose-fitting T-shirts up the back, and attach ties or Velcro to the neck. In bed the back can be left open so as to take advantage of the anti-bedsore mattress.

When the person with dementia starts going in for respite care, all their clothing must be named.

Clothing to avoid

This includes the following:
- no-longer-practical items such as feminine lacy silks
- flowered items – people with dementia may try to pick the flowers
- tights and pantyhose – they are not easy to put on
- tight garments that you have to pull over the head
- items with tight elastic, for example in socks
- open footwear that makes it easy to trip and fall.

Extras for saliva problems

If the person you are looking after begins to drool outside mealtime, make sure they have a large handkerchief available. Alternatively, tuck a large, easily washed polyester cloth under their chin. You could even sew tapes or Velcro on each corner of a hand towel to hang around their neck. (Some medications decrease saliva output, but take care: they can dry out mouths.)

Where to from here
- Chapter 8: Adapting the Home Environment, especially 'The bathroom'
- Chapter 21: Toileting
- Chapter 26: Moving into Full-time Care, especially 'Clothing in hospital'

Chapter 21

Toileting

Continence problems are very often part of dementia. If this happens to your charge, even if you feel you are managing, do enquire about their eligibility for assistance.

> After Alf had a stroke and developed dementia, no one told Kitty of all the help she was eligible for. She soldiered on for over nine years looking after him on her own. Uncomplaining and stoic, she adapted their home to his falls and foibles, and at night dealt with his incontinence by putting him in an enormous black plastic rubbish bag, tied at his waist – certainly not to be recommended, but the best she could do. She couldn't afford 'nappies', and didn't know that Alf could be assessed so that she could get them and other help free.

Ask your doctor or needs assessor for a referral to a community continence nurse, whose services may well be free. Helpful equipment is available through government agencies or your occupational therapist. Don't suffer – or let your charge suffer – in silence.

What is the cause?

Incontinence may become the bane of your existence, and it rules your life. It does not develop because of drinking too much, so do not deal with it by limiting drinks (see Chapter 19: Eating and Drinking, 'Getting enough fluids'). The cause of the incontinence may be treatable, or may at least be made more manageable.

Coordination, mobility

Many people with dementia do have some awareness and control of their muscles. They know when they want to go. However, they may be unable to manage their clothing in time.

> Several times while I have been visiting, Mum has had an 'accident' while going to the toilet. I do not believe this is an incontinence problem; more due to the fact that she cannot get her pants down quickly enough because of her restricted mobility.

If the person you are looking after has this problem and wears trousers or track pants, one way to make life easier is to undo the central front and back seams, cut the waistband there, hem those edges and sew Velcro in place of buttons down the front and back (making sure the Velcro will not rub against skin). Then all you or they have to do when they need to go to the toilet is pull open the front and/or back, enabling them to use the toilet or to remove and replace continence pads more easily.

Of course, the mobility problem may be more extensive: your charge knows when they want the toilet but can no longer walk. In this case, a 'shower-wheelchair-cum-commode' obtained from hospital or your occupational therapist could be their saviour.

Other people have difficulty aiming urine accurately. You may need to review the flooring and its coverings.

> A few years after Judy and Alan bought their house, Judy discovered the carpet at the base of the toilet had rotted. This was just before Alan was diagnosed with dementia, and his urine must have trickled down the outside of the bowl for quite some time. She replaced the carpet with vinyl.
>
> Much later, she put thick towels on the floor each night and left the light on for Alan to go to the bathroom on his own. If he fell and she had to get up to help him, she still had a better sleep than if she accompanied and monitored him (up to six times a night).

One way to improve a man's accuracy while urinating is to put a ping-pong ball in the bowl for him to aim at. It bobs up after every flush. You could also consider painting the walls in a bright colour, so that the white toilet pan stands out.

Saying what they need

In some cases, incontinence stems from a person's inability to communicate clearly, or the carer's failure to read the body language. Make sure day-care helpers and staff speak your charge's language, and are aware of their expressions – 'tinkle', 'take a leak', 'pee' and the like.

Getting lost may also be a factor. You can deal with this in numerous ways; you may even find a solution that's fun.

> Connie raided her family's games drawer for sticky, glittery funny faces. She stuck them on their bedroom carpet, in a track from Trevor's bed to the toilet, to help him find his way. She also wrote BATHROOM on a piece of white cardboard and stuck it on the door.

Night-time

Night-time brings darkness and increased disorientation. A light and closeness to the toilet will help.

> After over 30 years of marriage Mavis swapped her bed with Zac's, so that his king-sized single bed was closer to the toilet. Now he had a clear path for his night-time visits. She also bought a cheap battery-powered light. Placed on a bedside table, it took only a tap to turn it on and light him on his way.

Another possible night-time aid for men is a wide-necked bottle, placed near the bed in a bucket or a stable, high-sided waterproof container. (Sometimes a second bottle is needed.) Wash it out with a vinegar–water solution to stop smells.

Sleeping in a nightshirt makes using a bottle easier for men, and a short nightdress makes sitting on a toilet seat easier for women.

Toileting tips

- ✦ Your occupational therapist may be able to source grab rails to go next to the toilet and/or a toilet over-seat, adjustable to a comfortable height.
- ✦ Think about installing a hand bell in the bathroom so your charge can get your attention when necessary.
- ✦ If you occasionally have to help someone of the other gender to

use a public toilet, carry an OUT OF ORDER sign on a string to hang on the outside door handle while you are both inside.
+ Take a urine bottle, when you go out with a man with dementia, and know where the nearest toilets are.
+ Always carry dry underwear and/or incontinence pads when you go out together.

Protecting furnishings from urine

Before chair cushions get wet, think about placing vulnerable ones in large plastic bags inside a washable cover.

Before bed-wetting starts, replace an electric blanket with, perhaps, a thick sheepskin underlay, and cover the bottom sheet with a waterproof mattress protector. Buy two of the latter, so you can use a fresh one while washing the other.

> One carer found incontinence pads could not hold all his charge's urine. 'Buy a mattress protector,' he was advised, but nobody said where to put it. He put is on the mattress and washed sheets and the protector at least three times a week for months, until his support group finally told him it was meant to go on top of the bottom sheet. That was happiness – only one thing to wash instead of two.

Rather than buy a mattress protector you can create your own: fold a regular sheet in half lengthwise, put a plastic shield in between, and tuck the sheet in across the bed on both sides in a strategic place. (Choose plastic which won't crackle or rustle too much.)

Urinary protection your charge can wear
Continence pads and pants

Continence pads are the first line of defence against wet pants. They are much cheaper at supermarkets than at your pharmacist. However, a disability allowance may cover the cost of these if your charge is eligible. Once incontinence becomes the norm, the continence nurse can probably prescribe free pads. These may be pull-up, elasticised pants, with built-in medium protection, or more absorbent, nappy-like pads that are fastened with Velcro and easier to change.

If your charge wants to wear usual underwear over these pads, large disposable nappies made for toddlers are much easier to fit under knickers than the sticky-tab adult variety, especially when the wearer is restless while being changed. But remember they don't hold as much urine.

If you use two adult pads for extra protection, remove an inch-wide strip in the centre of the plastic band at the top of the inner pad, so that when this pad is saturated the excess spills over more easily into the outer layer. Sometimes, frustratingly, even this does not work for long and you just have to change the pads more often. If you are using two pads inside pull-up continence pants, buy the pants that split down the sides. They are the easiest to remove.

Have a supply of plastic bags close to where you change continence pads. Put the used pad into a plastic bag, tie that and toss it into your rubbish container: a metal-lidded pedal bin is most practical. (Buy one big enough to hold a day's worth of pads, with a washable bucket lined with a plastic bag inside. The bin's metal lid seems to control odours.)

External catheter for men

For men, an external catheter or urine-collecting device, known by nurses as a uri-sheath or uri-dome, is the second line of defence against wet beds at night. It consists of a rubber sheath on the penis, rather like a condom, with a long rubber tube at the end. This leads across the bed and into a container (bucket or large bottle) beside the bed.

If possible, start using it while the person with dementia can still appreciate having no more wet nightclothes and bedding. Initially they may want to put it on. Let them try once or twice to discover that you, perhaps, can do it more easily.

Internal catheter

The third line of defence for both sexes is a supra-pubic catheter: a rubber tube inserted directly into the bladder, under local anaesthetic in a doctor's surgery. The doctor's fee should cover the cost of this, plus the follow-up appointment. Once inserted, the management of it should be free. All the extra gear needed may come from a continence nurse, whom your charge should see every four, six or eight weeks to monitor progress.

During the day, the supra-pubic tube runs into a bag strapped to the wearer's upper leg. At bedtime the tube is taken out of this bag and directed into a large container by the bed. The container should be placed in another bucket or larger container in case it gets tipped over.

You can call the continence nurse if the tube gets blocked with bladder debris. This is not uncommon and is no cause for alarm; urine will find its way back down the urethra. Use continence pads until the nurse arrives. However, you may find that you can clear the blockage yourself by massaging the tube where the blockage is evident.

Perpetual bed-wetting

Both the external and supra-pubic tubes can be impractical if the wearer wanders at night-time, and sometimes even two incontinence pads worn by your charge are not enough to stem the flow in bed. When these solutions are impractical and bed-wetting eventually becomes a nightly event, you will need to devise a system to deal with it.

> Wallace always placed a folded thick towel on a chair near Thelma's side of their double bed. This was for her to sit on while he stripped away wet bedding. He placed clean bedding and pyjama pants within reach, too, so that he could remake the bed and wash and dry her with minimal delay. He became quite proud of the fact that all this could be done and they would be settling down to sleep again within five minutes.

Cleaning floors after urinary accidents

Keep a large supply of towels available. They don't have to be expensive ones, just absorbent. Wash and dry them immediately after use, ready for the next time.

On carpet

This system takes at least four towels for one accident. Adding lots of water helps banish the after-smell. You may also be able to buy products to remove urine stains and odours.

1. Mop up as much urine as possible with a towel, pushing in from the edge of the puddle so as not to enlarge the affected area.
2. Pour a small stream of cold water accurately around the outside edge of the puddle, to saturate only the affected area.
3. Mop up once more with a clean towel, pushing in from the outside in the same way.
4. Repeat as necessary.
5. Place a fresh towel over the wet patch and tread firmly on it all over, to soak up as much moisture as possible.
6. Remove that towel and place another dry one over the spot, folded as many times as possible to cover the spot and provide deep absorption.
7. Tread this firmly all over, leave in place and stamp on it frequently during the day, turning as it becomes damp. Replace if necessary.

On non-absorbent flooring
1. Put towels from your supply over the puddles to absorb the liquid.
2. Put the towels into a bucket and take them to the laundry tub for a sluice rinse.
3. Wash them in the washing machine, perhaps with a type of hygienic laundry rinse.
4. Clean the wet floor with a long-handled mop or sponge and bucket of warm water. Keep your charge clear of the area until it is dry.
5. Buy two of these mops. Keep one permanently in the bathroom and one in the kitchen, with a spare mophead in reserve.

Lack of bowel control
Try to identify toilet need signals, and accommodate old habits. Some people have always read the morning paper while sitting on the toilet, so keep a newspaper or other disposable reading material handy – it may keep them happy and help them do the job.

Assist when needed. You may find that the person you are looking after cannot wipe themselves clean after defecating, and underpants get soiled at a great rate. Get your charge used to bending over while you use the toilet paper for them.

Skin-cleaning tips

+ Consider using baby wipes for little clean-ups or finishing touches, and skin moisturisers for long-term protection.
+ Baby oil on toilet paper helps remove faeces caked on the skin more easily, avoiding abrasion.
+ For massive messes on your charge's skin, use muslin, which can be bought by the metre, or use warm, soapy paper towels gently and repeatedly, until the area looks clean. Finish off with baby wipes or hand wipes, apply baby oil, moisturiser if necessary, and pat dry with soft toilet paper or fabric.

Poor coordination

Increasing difficulties with coordination will eventually mean they can't position their bottom on the seat.

> Bruce knew when he wanted to relieve himself but couldn't back himself down onto the toilet seat. Going on his own, he sometimes squatted sideways to the toilet bowl and deposited his motion on the floor.
>
> Once, when Alison was there, he went into the bathroom, advanced on the toilet, pulled his pants down and grasped the over-seat handles on either side. His expression was determined ('I'm going to get the best of you this time'), but he could not turn around.
>
> Alison tried to pick up his feet and move them, but his Parkinsonism kept them rigid. She tried to pick him up bodily, but he was too heavy. She asked him to let the handles go, turn around and see who was standing in the doorway, but he knew she was kidding him.
>
> They both wanted the same outcome but could not find a solution until Alison said, 'Brucie, let's dance.'
>
> He turned around, looking quizzical, reached out and took her in his arms, and they waltzed a few steps around the bathroom until she had steered him into position. Just that once everything went perfectly.

Cleaning up after bowel accidents

When bowels move unexpectedly, start your hygiene procedures. Have a box of light, cheap rubber gloves always nearby, and put gloves on before you clean up both your charge and the mess.

First take the person with dementia away from the scene, wash them thoroughly and change clothing as necessary. Settle them in a comfortable spot and ask them to stay there while you clear up.

Carefully clean the floor, toilet seat, flush handle, basin and taps – all the area where the accident happened, and anything that could have been contaminated. You don't want either of you becoming the next tummy-bug victim.

Put all soiled clothing and cloths in a special bucket, sluice them (in a tub or, sometimes, in several toilet flushes, holding on tightly) and machine-wash them on their own. Supermarkets offer some laundry products that claim an antibacterial effect. These seem quite effective in maintaining hygiene. Be on the lookout for any irritation to the skin. Skin sensitivity can be exacerbated by detergents, and by the thinness of skin in older people, as well as by frequent contact with urine because of incontinence.

For constant bowel incontinence

Once the person with dementia reaches the stage of constant bowel incontinence, keep a special cleaning kit at the ready:

- ✦ rubber gloves
- ✦ several washing cloths (such as old kitchen cloths) and old towels for drying
- ✦ bowls or buckets to hold warm water
- ✦ a roll of toilet paper and sheets of newspaper
- ✦ a special knife or spatula
- ✦ different types of brushes – toilet, scrubbing or bottle brushes – for diverse contaminated spaces
- ✦ carpet shampoo (find out which is the best) and disinfectant (optional)
- ✦ anything else your initiative suggests.

Twelve steps to remove soft faeces from carpet

Put all your gear at the scene of the accident and get to work as cheerfully as possible.

1. Put on the gloves and put warm water in several containers beside the mess.
2. Kneel down and spread the newspaper to one side, plus toilet paper.
3. Carefully scoop up the faeces with your special implement, and wipe it into a bunch of toilet paper in your other hand. Place this on the newspaper. Repeat until you have removed most of the faeces.
4. Roll up the newspaper and put it away, ready for the rubbish bin.
5. Wet your scrubbing brush using warm water from one container, and remove the remaining surface faeces by scrubbing the area from the outside to the centre, trying not to extend the area too much.
6. Wipe off with a rag.
7. Rinse the brush and repeat.
8. Put a few drops of carpet shampoo on to the spot and scrub with clean water from a second container, working again from the outside to the centre.
9. Remove the lather with another rag, soak the area with clean water from the third container and mop up again with more rags.
10. Repeat until most of the lather has disappeared.
11. Place a clean towel over the patch and treat as you would a urine spill.
12. Open windows to allow smells to disperse ('air fresheners' may only make this unpleasant smell worse).

Coping with constipation

Many, but not all, people with Parkinson's dementia develop constipation because the usual movements of the intestines slow down along with the body's other muscles. It is common among people who have other dementias too, especially if their dementia is advanced and they spend much of the day immobile.

The normal number of bowel movements ranges – from two to three daily, to one every two or three days. As long as your charge feels comfortable, don't worry.

With no movements for four-plus days, however, they may feel bloated or uncomfortable, and their anal area may be hard and bulging. They may also have a faecal leak, due to the bowel's heroic efforts to get things moving by producing extra lubrication (the stool doesn't move; only some surface faecal matter emerges, looking and smelling like a small, loose motion). In either case intervention is called for. Your doctor may prescribe oral or rectal medication.

Another reason for constipation may be medication, including tranquillisers, antidepressants, painkillers (analgesics – nothing to do with 'anal'!). Certain foods can also be to blame.

For regular bowel movements

Give your charge a balanced diet of high-fibre foods, including wholemeal breads and pastas, cereals, pulses and dried fruits. Some people need different quantities from others, so check with your dietician. You can add bran flakes to cereals, stewed fruit and puddings, and offer plenty of fresh fruit and vegetables, for necessary vitamins.

A continence nurse can also indicate the foods that cause trouble with bowel motions, and your journal can record which produce good or regrettable results.

Having lots of fluids (not all teas and coffees and alcohol!) helps keep the bowels moving. Perhaps try two full glasses of water or some other neutral liquid your charge likes, between meals. Plenty of exercise also helps.

The balancing act

Continence and toileting issues demand much of the carer: as well as looking out for accidents, you need to be alert for anything that suggests a medical problem. As with a long period of constipation, frequent loose stools in your charge always need to be investigated. They may be signs of other treatable conditions.

Likewise, double incontinence can have other causes apart from dementia: infections, cancer of the bowel or bladder, bladder or kidney stones, prostate problems, hernia, prolapse of womb or rectum, diabetes, irritable bowel syndrome or diverticulitis, dehydration, immobility, faecal impaction ... your charge may keep you on your toes.

Sometimes the dementia journey offers unpleasant surprises, and it can be hard not to feel shocked or repulsed.

> Harry had been wandering around the house all morning, but was now sitting at the table playing dominoes or something. His carer suddenly realised that the dominoes were still in the games cupboard. There were lots of interesting little shapes on the table – and what his carer thought was a sculptured banana proved on inspection to be horribly 'or something'.

If your charge gives you such surprise packages, try not to become a gibbering wreck. Do your best never to display impatience or disapproval. If they have no awareness of the trouble they are causing, they will be very upset to have you growling at them for 'nothing'.

Times like this really prove the worth of a support group: a bunch of people with whom you can let off steam and laugh, and who will identify with your experience.

> Joan wearily told her support group of Greer's new use for their clothes basket – as a urinal. She was rather put out when someone quipped, 'Well, that's a very absorbent place to go, isn't it? My Pat goes in much less suitable places,' and the others laughed uproariously.
>
> On another occasion Joan told the group of finding squares of used toilet paper in the soiled clothes basket. She was amazed to discover that most of them had had the same experience.

Where to from here

✦ Chapter 8: Adapting the Home Environment
✦ Chapter 9: Managing Difficult Behaviour
✦ Chapter 11: Independence and Safety
✦ Chapter 19: Eating and Drinking, especially 'Getting enough fluids'
✦ Chapter 20: Showering and Dressing
✦ Chapter 22: Wandering
✦ Chapter 23: Hallucinations, Delusions and Delirium

Chapter 22

Wandering

Ten reasons why people wander

Some people with dementia are compulsive, long-distance wanderers; others simply like to pace aimlessly, indoors or outdoors. The following are some common reasons for those behaviours, and suggestions for dealing with them:

1. Curiosity, boredom or restlessness – have more for your person with dementia to do (see Chapter 17: Entertainment).
2. Need for more exercise – arrange a daily walk with someone, or find a safe, enclosed area where they can exercise freely (see Chapter 16: Exercise).
3. Loneliness – get more company in for them or take them to day care.
4. Looking for the children, their sibling, or others – keep family photo albums out.
5. Seeking a familiar routine or profession, such as going to church, bowls or the office – reintroduce elements of a familiar routine.
6. Disorientation, for example they don't think they are at home or are looking for their childhood home – offer them their life book to browse through.
7. Hunger or thirst – give easier access to snacks.
8. Avoiding hubbub – reduce clutter, noise and worrying aspects around them.
9. Wondering what time it is – have large analogue or digital clocks within view.

10. Wanting to see better, if they are in dimly lit surroundings – use stronger light bulbs, spend time in rooms with larger windows.

Use your powers of deduction

Often the person you are looking after may not be able to tell you in words why they are wandering. If it happens at the same time each day, try to work out – using their life book – where they think they should be and what they should be doing.

If it is usually about 10 am when they set off, perhaps they think they should be going to work or shopping? Consider dropping what you are doing and walking or driving with them to the shops to make a few purchases.

Wanderings at around 4.30 pm may indicate that they feel it is time they started leaving work, or getting a meal together, so go for a walk or start them on setting the table or helping prepare the meal.

If it is later in the evening, your charge may believe it is time to put children to bed or tidy the house. Ask them to turn down some beds, get a book or two for bedtime stories, plump up cushions and so forth.

Precautions

You may need to take some precautions, especially at night-time, although it would be sad if the person you are caring for felt like a prisoner.

Put car keys away, as wandering isn't always on foot. If night-time is a problem, leave lights on in the house and fence off stairs they could fall down.

Preparing exits

A bell that jingles when an exit door is opened could be a useful signal to you as caregiver, if it does not drive you crazy in the meantime. An alternative is to attach a baby or toddler monitor to your charge. These, available in children's and electronics stores, let you hear the sounds made nearby or, in some cases, set off a beeper if the person goes more than 10 or 20 metres away.

As a deterrent, you can lock or otherwise deactivate doors to the outside world. Child-proof doorknob covers, also available at children's stores, prevent knobs from being turned (but they are not easy for carers with arthritis).

Consider using slide bolts at the top and/or bottom of doors to the outside, and install unfamiliar locks on doors and gates. You can install deadlocks that require a key for exit and entrance, but make sure they can be quickly unlocked in case of fire. Lock all exits at night.

> Tony woke up one night to find that Martha wasn't beside him in bed. He leapt up and had just reached the bedroom door when Martha appeared, quietly coming down the hall. Apparently she had been up to the local shops (in her nightgown), looking for an old tennis friend. Tony bought a latch and padlock the next day.

Identification

An identity bracelet for your charge should show their name, address and phone number. Blood group and allergies could be considered, too. Special bracelets for the latter can be obtained from some dementia-related organisations.

On pieces of card, write out your own name (specifying that you are the carer) and phone numbers – work, sports club, mobile, and so on – and those of other family members. Put one in the pocket of each garment the person with dementia might wear. Use indelible pen (not ballpoint), but remember to take the cards out when washing clothes.

Let the police, local shops and neighbours know if your charge begins to wander. Sew reflector tape on clothing, to help police car headlights locate your wanderer and improve safety at night. Keep an unwashed piece of their clothing for tracker dogs to sniff, and copies of a photograph (a good likeness) to hand out if necessary.

Day and night

Wandering can happen during the day as well as at night, so plan your precautions with this in mind.

> Greer was able to spend the day alone at home while Joan was at work – until he wandered for the first time. He'd called a taxi 'to take him to the dentist' and was rather vague when telling the taxi

driver where to go. They had gone round and round the city during his confusion.

More than $100 later, in some desperation, the taxi driver took Greer to his own dentist. This man recognised the problem, eventually found Joan's phone number in Greer's pocket, and phoned her, asking what to do. Greer had nothing wrong with his teeth, no dental appointment and no money. Joan just had to find what was now a $120 taxi fare.

Instant reactions

When wandering happens, you can react instantly in several ways. See which work for you.

If the person you are caring for tries to leave the house, don't try to stop them physically. This may result in aggression and hurt, or emotional distress (on both sides). If they can't be persuaded to come back inside, go with them on their walk, or take them for a drive round the block, or let them go – and follow, to make sure they come home safely. Even in the middle of the night, a few minutes of this are better than the hours of distress (and possible injury) that can result from trying to stop them doing what they wish.

If you see that your charge is out and it is too late to try the strategies above, leave the house unobtrusively, note which direction they are going and try to meet them 'by chance'. Grab a bus fare as you leave, as many a person with dementia has hopped on to a bus, with sublime disregard for the fare and even their destination.

When you catch up with them, walk a distance with them before, surreptitiously, steering them back home. Alternatively, give them a hug, lead them to a safe place and spend time with them until they seem settled again.

Balancing risks and rights

Restrictions on wandering are usually for the peace of mind of the carer, rather than the safety of the person at risk. Consider how much right a person with dementia has to live their own life as they wish, even if it may involve risk.

Usually, a lost person is only temporarily mislaid. They will often find their way to a familiar place, though the carer may have some worrying moments until they are located.

Sarah, who had been in a regular dementia support group with Connie for two years, rushed up to Connie and Trevor at the supermarket. 'Have you seen Tom?' she blurted out. 'He was with me two minutes ago and now I can't find him!' Ever helpful, Trevor said, 'We'll go look for him.' Ever pragmatic, Connie said, 'But we've never met him. We don't know what he looks like.'

That evening Connie phoned Sarah to find out how the situation ended. 'Oh, you wouldn't believe it,' Sarah said, laughing. 'From the supermarket I went to the police and then home, and there was Tom, sitting in the sun. He'd wanted to go home, and found his way from three miles away. He's not as demented as I thought!'

Good Samaritans

Be aware, too, that the wider community includes people of goodwill who will generally intervene if they find a lost soul.

The specialist told Penelope that Richard needed to feel independent and should still be playing golf. Against her better judgement, Penelope took him out to the links the next day, arranged a time to pick him up, then drove off uneasily. That was the last she saw of him until late that night when, after hours of anguish, she answered the phone to a woman who said, 'I think I've got something that belongs to you.'

Richard had left the golf course and walked several kilometres back to where they now lived, but then kept going. He had actually nearly reached the next little town 17 kilometres away when he tumbled into a ditch.

A passer-by who pulled him out recognised his condition, and when Richard told him that he lived across the harbour (where he used to live), the rescuer took him all the way to the wharf and put him on the next ferry. The man then phoned a nurse he knew, who lived on the other side, and asked her to meet Richard, warning her about the dementia.

Richard was nowhere in sight by the time this woman reached the ferry landing but she eventually picked him up, still plodding along, a few kilometres further on. She could see dementia in his eyes and dehydration in his face, so bought him a large orange drink, searched his clothing while he gulped it down, and located the piece of paper with his personal details, which Penelope always put in a pocket when he went out.

The woman rang Penelope immediately, drove to the vehicular ferry, crossed the harbour and drove Richard all the way home, arriving just before midnight. While Penelope was almost collapsing with relief, Richard was charmingly unfazed and grateful, and insisted on paying for the bottle of orange.

In care

If you find your charge at day care in a chair that has a table clipped on the front, to keep them there and prevent them from wandering, ask whether this is really necessary. Restrictions are not meant to be part of the caring environment. It is best to choose a place with a secured perimeter, one where they can move about as they wish. It is illegal to restrict someone, or to sedate them deeply, unless they are in 'protective custody', in prison, in a mental hospital, or a danger to someone else.

Where to from here

- Chapter 8: Adapting the Home Environment
- Chapter 9: Managing Difficult Behaviour, especially 'Sundowning or twilighting'
- Chapter 10: Wider Support and Self-care
- Chapter 11: Independence and Safety
- Chapter 12: Feelings
- Chapter 13: Communication
- Chapter 17: Entertainment
- Chapter 23: Hallucinations, Delusions and Delirium
- Chapter 24: Aggression
- Chapter 25: Choosing Full-time Care, especially 'Use of restraints'

Chapter 23

Hallucinations, Delusions and Delirium

At times you may be astonished by the person you are looking after. They seem to live in a completely different world from you, and they really believe what they are experiencing or whatever conclusion they have come to. They may be misinterpreting what they see, hallucinating, or being paranoid.

Not all people with dementia have these experiences or deluded beliefs, but many do. You can try to explain to them that what they are experiencing or believing is not real. But if you accept their view, you will avoid arguments that can take up a lot of your time and that you are unlikely to win in any case.

Paranoia

Even people who are well can feel suspicious now and then about particular events or people in their lives. Ideally – and often – they investigate, think things through and come to a rational conclusion about whether their suspicion is based in fact. A person with paranoia, however, does not think things through and has firm beliefs that are delusional. These often involve blame, jealousy or a sense of persecution.

When someone with dementia develops paranoia, the part of their brain that makes judgements and separates facts from fiction may be damaged. They may also be struggling to make sense of events and their environment, due to an overwhelming symptom of their dementia: forgetfulness.

Hallucinations, Delusions and Delirium

An inability to remember means that people with dementia must constantly rediscover and reinterpret the world around them. If they already feel they lack control of their life, for instance if they live reluctantly in a nursing home, it is easy for paranoia to develop.

> Phoebe accused her daughter of taking three $50 notes from under the mattress, despite her daughter having been away in Spain for a month. Phoebe forgot she hid them in her shoes.

You could confront Phoebe with the fact that her daughter was overseas when the money 'disappeared'. This will not restore her sense of calm and control, however; nor will it bring back the other thing that's missing – the money. A better idea may be to help Phoebe look for the money she's lost.

Hallucinations and misinterpretations

Hallucinations involve perceiving things that (to everybody else) are not present, rather than mistaking an existing thing for something else. They are mostly visual, but may also include touch, hearing or smell. People with Lewy body dementia, in particular, often have hallucinations – though they can occur in other dementias.

Misinterpretations and hallucinations alike can require carers to have a sense of humour and an open mind. One common scenario involves a long-time spouse suddenly finding they have a rival:

> Janine was nearly asleep when Jeffrey turned over to her in bed and said, 'Oh there you are. I thought you were on this side. I've got another woman here.'
>
> Janine thought fast. How should she respond? 'Oh, really?' she replied. 'What's her name?'
>
> Jeffrey turned away and said to the empty space beside him, 'What's your name?' He turned back to Janine and said, 'She says her name is Bessie.' And from that night onwards, three people shared the bed.

◆

> Judy and Alan were starting dinner when Judy remembered the potatoes she'd left on the stove. She told Alan and went into the kitchen. When she returned with them, Alan looked up with his

charming smile (which he kept for visitors) and said, 'Hullo. Who are you? Did you meet my wife in the kitchen?' Judy said, 'No. I'll go out and see if she's still there.' She went back in, stood a few moments then returned. Alan looked up with his normal deadpan face and said, 'Did you see that strange woman? She looked very like you. She went looking for you.'

'Then I'll go and look for her,' said Judy, fascinated. Again she stood out of sight before returning. 'Well, hullo again,' Alan said with his winning smile. 'Judy went to find you. Did you meet her this time?'

Judy thought it was time to stop the charade. 'Alan, darling, there is no other woman. It was all me. That's why she looked like me! It was another of your hallucinations, but much more complicated than usual.'

Alan looked at her blankly, made no comment and started to eat. But all through the meal, he addressed comments to the unknown woman, who now sat opposite Judy.

Behaving as though you believe your charge and acting your way out the other side may be the simplest response to their perception, even if initially you feel rather silly.

Linda took a mug of tea in to Earl, her father. He held out his hand: 'Take all these threads off my fingers, Linnie,' he said. 'They're sticking there and I can't hold the mug until I get rid of them.' So Linda put down the mug and carefully wiped each of Earl's fingers clean – of nothing. 'Thanks, dear. That's done the trick,' he said and took his mug.

When your person with dementia sees something that isn't there, or isn't what they think it is, it catches their attention. They ask you to share it. Usually they are just intrigued because it seems unusual.

You could ask them to describe in detail what they are seeing or experiencing. Say, 'I know you see/feel/smell it. You tell me what's there. I can't sense it. Is it upsetting you?' Try to see with their eyes or feel with their other senses. Avoid confrontation. Their response may surprise you, and it may explain their actions. They may be annoyed, worried or uncomfortable, but usually their hallucinations or delusions won't upset

Hallucinations, Delusions and Delirium

them. You may be more upset. There is no need to be – unless they are. Sometimes, an unreal perception that bothers your charge may call for a completely fantastical solution.

When Barbara heard Jack get up unusually early one morning, she asked where he was going. Jack told her there was a man kneeling beside his bed, and he was making faces at him and wouldn't go away. So he was getting out and leaving him there. His wife called him back and tried to persuade him he was imagining things before, finally, deciding to try another tack. 'Would you like me to call the matron and ask her to get rid of the man beside your bed?' she asked.

'Can you do that?' he said, standing in the doorway.

'Of course,' she replied, and she picked up the phone, pretended to dial a number and acted her way through the following conversation. 'Matron, this is Barbara. I'm calling to ask you to tell that man kneeling beside Jack's bed to go away. He's not very happy with it.... Okay? ... Yes, thanks very much.'

Jack looked totally relieved. 'Thanks, you always know what to do.' He got into bed and promptly fell asleep.

If safety is a concern, you may need to be assertive and act decisively to stop behaviour that is based on a misinterpretation or hallucination.

Earl grabbed Linda's lower arm in a vice-like grip, and dragged her out of his room and into the passage.

'What are you doing, Dad?' she protested.

'I've got to get this chair to the dining room,' he muttered, pulling her along.

Linda said gently: 'Dad, I'm not a chair. I'm Linda. Please let me go.' He took no notice. Linda resisted. She tried a firmer voice: 'No, Dad, let me go. I'm not a chair.' Gazing fixedly ahead, he still ignored her and dragged her along very roughly.

Linda put on the commanding voice she used when her children ran riot: 'Earl, you are a naughty boy! Let me go!' At that moment either he thought she was his mother, or his forward momentum got out of control. He let go and collapsed on the carpet. Shaking, she raced off to call a staff member and left Earl to their ministrations.

It is easier to avoid misinterpretations than to avoid hallucinations. A carer can do this by changing the thing that the person with dementia misinterprets. In one case, the person with dementia imagined flowers in the patterned curtains in his room were people, and carried on conversations with them. If the people he saw bothered him, or if he had real-life roommates who found the conversations intolerable, his carer could have replaced the curtains with plain ones, and his 'people' would vanish.

Poor lighting and visual disturbances caused by cataracts, scratched spectacles or other problems with eyesight, can cause some misinterpretations by people with dementia. These can usually be dealt with, making life less disturbing – or possibly even slightly less interesting – for the people concerned.

Delirium

Delirium is a mental disturbance that is usually marked by suddenly upset behaviour, and alertness fluctuates over the course of a day. Your charge may be lucid one moment and drowsy or very confused the next. They may stumble in their speech, not know where they are, see or hear things that are not there, appear very frightened, or be restless or aggressive – or they may sit abnormally quietly.

If such symptoms appear suddenly, get to a doctor as soon as possible. These are not part of your charge's normal dementia, and their cause needs diagnosis and treatment. Generally the delirium won't last long once this is done.

Delirium has many possible causes. A frequent one is an infection in the body, and the cellulitis described here is typical:

> Trevor seemed extra confused. His hand had swelled up to twice its size overnight and red streaks were shooting up his arm. Connie took him straight to their doctor who immediately responded, 'Cellulitis. I'll alert the hospital. Take him there right now.'
>
> That was the last Connie saw of 'her' Trevor for eight days, as he lay attached to bottles and drips, fighting fever and infection. He became a stranger. He didn't know her when she visited, and refused to be fed, even by her.

The registrar on duty warned her that Trevor might never know her again, that this was the way of dementia with delirium. Luckily she found on the ninth day that she hadn't lost him completely: some of the old Trevor came home when he was discharged; but some of him remained behind.

Medications can also cause delirium. In the following story, a carer's vigilance helped distinguish between her husband's irreversible dementia and much more treatable delirium:

Alan, home again after a spell in hospital and sitting comfortably in his usual armchair, began gnawing at his left fore-finger. 'There's not much meat on this chicken bone,' he complained to Judy.
He seemed suddenly to be completely unaware of where he was and the reality around him. Alarmed that he might do himself real damage, Judy took him and his hospital discharge papers straight up to their doctor's surgery where they were given an immediate appointment.
'Oh-ho,' said the doctor, as he skim-read the hospital notes. 'I see they have given him a new drug. That'll be the cause of his delirium. It's a complete enemy of the regular medication he's on.'

Where to from here

- Chapter 7: Dealing with Health Professionals
- Chapter 8: Adapting the Home Environment
- Chapter 9: Managing Difficult Behaviour
- Chapter 13: Communication
- Chapter 15: Maintaining Health
- Chapter 22: Wandering
- Chapter 24: Aggression

Chapter 24

Aggression

There may be times when even the gentlest personality undergoes a drastic transformation. The person you are caring for may, to your astonishment, lose control, become physically violent, hit out and throw things around. Or they may talk loudly and abusively, flail legs and arms uncontrollably, have a tantrum or collapse in tears.

There is no saying whether or not this will happen in your case, but it is such a common occurrence with dementia – and the stimuli for aggression can be so unexpected – that you would be well advised to be mentally prepared.

Influences and immediate causes

In general, violence is a response to a perceived threat; or an attempt to control someone or something, or a result of frustration. In someone with dementia, aggressive behaviour is usually influenced by medications, the environment, what the person was doing at the time, or upsetting communication with others (including the carer).

The immediate, specific causes of aggression tend to be situations or feelings that can crowd in on someone with dementia. Those listed below can be categorised, broadly, as:

- being overwhelmed
- a sense of powerlessness
- a medical problem.

In everyday life, people who have no additional challenges deal with these matter-of-factly, or with humour or irritation. To someone with dementia, however, they can be extremely upsetting and lead to mayhem.

Sometimes it may not be clear what prompted an outburst, or there may be more than one cause. For instance, John in the story below may be frustrated by a simple task (being overwhelmed), and very likely feels insulted by being treated like a child (a sense of powerlessness).

> John, one of the quietest, gentlest and most charming of men, developed Alzheimer's in his retirement. He was easy most of the time, but then began sometimes unexpectedly flying into awful rages when Dinah, his wife, tried to get him ready for bed. He would have a real tantrum, fling his pyjamas in her face and storm out of the room, swearing and shouting at her. She would be frightened.
>
> At first she tried to insist that he change for bed but, as weeks went by and these outbursts continued, she felt 'peace at any price' and left him to sleep in his clothes. By the morning, after one of these rampages, he would be his usual lovely self. Awakening, he would turn over to her and say with a smile, 'Well, how are you today, sweetie?'

Being overwhelmed

Your charge may now be very sensitive and react negatively after:
- having to endure loud noises from radio, television, traffic or crowds of people
- being pestered with 'Why?' or 'What?' questions
- being asked to do something they now can't manage, even a simple task such as doing up buttons
- receiving complicated directions or instructions
- becoming very tired from insufficient sleep
- unexpected physical contact.

A sense of powerlessness

From your charge's perspective, the way they have been treated or what is happening to them may seem unfair, and they may feel powerless. They may:

- feel left out and insecure while becoming aware of their decline
- have had toileting accidents or be in uncomfortable clothes
- have to put up with a new or unsuitable caregiver
- have had their schedule or routine changed
- have felt insulted by being treated like a child or imbecile
- have been reprimanded or had someone argue with them.

The following common scenario features someone whose dementia has advanced another stage (a medical problem):

> After several years of peacefully being cared for by Wallace, Thelma unexpectedly screamed and viciously attacked him one night as he began to unbutton her blouse while getting her ready for bed. He was very shaken and didn't know what to do, so fled, leaving her yelling in the bedroom. He cleaned his teeth, put on his own pyjamas and waited. After a while the screaming stopped. He let silence last for a few minutes then poked his nose cautiously round the bedroom door. Thelma was standing where he had left her, looking forlorn. He spoke to her gently, she turned to him, smiled, and let him undress her and put on her pyjamas with no more fuss.
>
> Over the next year Thelma attacked him at bedtime every two or three nights. Wallace never knew when it would happen and never resisted; he simply went away and did something else until he heard her quieten down. He worked out that she had reached the stage where she didn't recognise him all the time, and resisted 'the strange man' who was trying to undress her.

A medical problem

Another immediate cause of your charge's outburst could be discomfort that has a particular medical basis:

- physical discomfort through pain, fever, illness, faecal blockage, dehydration
- side-effects from medications
- problems seeing or hearing properly, leading them to misinterpret events, conversations, sights or sounds – perhaps having hallucinations or delusions

- the beginning of a severe infection
- having their condition progress another step, or being affected by a looming illness
- knuckling under due to depression.

Aggression can be the result of deterioration in the part of the brain that inhibits antisocial impulses. Some forms of dementia, such as fronto-temporal dementia, involve more aggression than others.

In the following case, hospital staff called in the home carer to calm their patient, who seemed to be suffering from a side-effect of a new medicine:

> After Edward's heart attack, doctors at the intensive care ward continued his Parkinson's tablets but added other medications, such as a blood thinner. One medication did not agree with him and he went on a rampage, whipping out his drips and storming round the ward.
>
> Someone phoned his wife. She agreed to come straight away, but suggested that, in the meantime, they read him the morning paper's business section. When she arrived, he was in bed again, being read to, hooked up to his drips and electrodes, successfully sedated and blissfully back where he had spent most of his life, absorbing the day's business ups and downs, rampage forgotten.

Another hospital story has the person with dementia suffering acute infection as well as injuries:

> Colin was admitted to hospital after a fall. The strange hospital surroundings and his fever, grazes, cellulitis and pneumonia pushed Colin into a constant aggressive state. The second day Gwenda arrived to find four large orderlies sitting on him and another injecting a sedative.
>
> In the tense two weeks that followed, Colin was forcibly kept in bed behind raised bars with a special attendant. Gwenda was often called to the hospital late at night to settle him during his extra-aggressive sundowning spells.

Ways to respond

Even you might erupt if you could not say, 'I don't want to do this because...', and so found yourself being forced to do something. It is vital that you don't ever punish. And don't try to restrain your charge if they become aggressive or agitated, unless they are attacking someone else. Give them space. Don't whisper or laugh: this may inflame the aggression.

If you feel safe and decide to stay, be gentle and matter of fact.

Try to sense the feelings behind the person's words or actions. Facial expressions and non-verbal body language can often tell you. So can a good knowledge of their life experiences and their personality.

Name the feelings you sense they have, and show with warmth that you accept them as normal. Show that you accept your charge as the person they are, and that their upset is only to be expected. Hopefully, they will be soothed by your acceptance.

Reassure the person with dementia. Reassure yourself, too: you are coping with an organic brain disease. Your charge is not deliberately being violent, stubborn or obtuse.

Position yourself in front of the person and at the same eye level, gaining their attention. Speak as you would like to be spoken to yourself.

Appear relaxed, calm, smiling; try not to show fear. Use the person's name and simple, familiar words in statements that are easy to understand. Speak slowly and clearly in a low-pitched voice (a high-pitched voice can make an angry person worse).

Apologise for any way you may have upset them. Give them a hug, pat their back or hold their hand (as long as they don't sense this as a restraint or inappropriate closeness). If the person needs help, try not to step in too quickly. Let them do things their way, even if it means you help them put their singlet on over their shirt.

Talk with your charge about their aggression, putting words to their feelings (if you are positive you have pinpointed them) or giving 'I' messages of your own (see Chapter 12: Feelings, '"I" messages'). If you, too, find yourself starting to become annoyed, admit that you are both getting nowhere. Leave the scene quickly if you might be hurt.

> The group at day care was enjoying the afternoon sunshine while Flora, their attendant, took them through the simple quiz they always had on Fridays. Elmer, a newcomer, sat quietly with the others at the table while his wife Dawn sat unobtrusively in a corner of the room.

Suddenly Elmer shouted, pushed his chair back, stood up and swiped all the crockery near him on to the floor, then charged off in a rage.

Dawn followed him, while Flora calmed the others down and began to clear up. When Dawn caught up with Elmer he was looking at freedom through the plate glass of the front door. 'Oh, Elmer, you hated that quiz, didn't you?' his wife said.

'Silly bloody stuff it was,' he muttered. 'As though we want to be buggered about with all that garbage.'

'Yes,' Dawn agreed, 'it seems like a bloody waste of time, doesn't it? Your first day here and you're fed up!'

'Too right,' he agreed. 'I didn't want to come here. They made me. I want to be at home. Not f–ing here.'

'Yes. Home's the best place, Elmer. I look after you there, don't I?'

'Yes, you're my old girl. You've got awful arthritis. I've got this and you've got that, but I don't know why you made me come here once a week.'

'It was the family, dear,' Dawn said, 'I'm getting on a bit and they can't have you for the day now. They've gone off to live in England with their new baby. You know, they're going to live where you used to, in Gloucester. You were brought up in Gloucester.'

With his mind on another subject, Elmer simmered down. He and Dawn sat on the nearby armchairs and reminisced about their family, England and Gloucester, before he joined the others for Happy Hour. The calamity was apparently forgotten; but Elmer was excused from the quiz after that.

Dawn's approach was first class and her method of communicating effective. She identified Elmer's feelings, accepted them and introduced a new subject, and this settled him down.

Try a new beginning

Slow everything down to their pace. Stay interested and friendly. Once the aggressive one feels understood and has calmed down, choose some comfortable way for you both to make a new beginning. If you have to ask questions, only ask ones that need 'Yes' or 'No' answers.

Bring up an interesting subject to distract them and take their mind off the trouble. Talk cheerfully, be sociable and generally chatty – about family, their health and doings, or any other subjects easy for you both. Use humour with them, but not at them. Praise achievement.

Perhaps suggest a well-liked food or activity: you could read to them from a favourite book or the newspaper; start a favourite song, hoping they may join in; recall an old family story to get them talking.

Other options include walking around the house, garden or street (taking your companion's arm if appropriate); or turning on the television, the radio or some music.

Make sure, however, that they don't feel such activities are dismissing their unhappiness. These alternatives involve, of course, knowledge of the person's interests and personality. Now you have to remember these in an emergency!

Catastrophic reactions

When a person with dementia is grossly overloaded, they may erupt and whirl into astounding, uncontrollable behaviour. They may pull at your glasses, push or punch you, or even take a swing at you.

When you can, try to imagine what it's like for them to be so restricted all the time. They are still them inside, but they can't get out, and they don't think you, or the person looking after them, understands.

In public

If your charge erupts like this at the shops, a concert or a party, you can't hold them up under one arm and move away, as with a child having a tantrum. Instead, accept that they are feeling wild. Don't argue or reprimand. Empathise with understanding and reassurance. ('Ooh, this is all too much. Let's get away from here.')

Try to remove them from whatever public place they are in, in a quiet, unhurried manner. People noticing will just be glad it is not they who have to cope. A strong, sincere statement such as 'You are very upset and

I want to help you' may defuse the situation. Take their hand as you lead them away, or just touch them affectionately (if they don't mind being touched), and point to something or hand them something to distract them. (This is preferable to giving your charge drugs, which can quieten them completely but may have harmful side-effects.)

If these ways of defusing a situation have no effect, it may be better to ignore the person creating the scene and walk away, especially if you are the one who caused their fury. But you need to make sure, somehow, that other people nearby don't get involved or hurt.

Comfort yourself by realising that the angry or threatening behaviours are not always personal attacks. They are often just symptoms of the dementia.

At home

If a catastrophic reaction occurs in the home, you may have more resources on hand to help you respond, but there may be no other people you can call on.

Don't force the person to do something they are resisting. When they react in an extreme way, stay calm. If you panic, they may become far worse.

Try to avoid sudden moves such as jumping up or running behind a table. Reduce any nearby noise or confusion, such as that caused by high-spirited grandchildren, and if possible remove your charge from a distressing situation such as a complaining neighbour.

Sit on a sofa and pat it, suggesting that the person sit down beside you. Hold their hand or offer them a pillow to punch. If they don't like to be touched, leave the room or sit quietly at a safe distance. Eventually, and cautiously, distract your charge into an activity they can easily do and usually enjoy, for instance, eating or music.

Restrain the person only if absolutely necessary and you have help. Remember that it took four orderlies to subdue one patient (see 'A medical problem', above). The bad dreams of the man discussed below were a nightmare for his carer, but it may not have been a good idea to grab him when he was half-asleep:

> He has terrible nightmares and I have to sleep in the same bed so that I can get hold of his pyjamas before he throws himself out of bed. I have to hold him the best way I can, but he becomes violent and has hurt me many times. Occasionally I have to phone for my son when I cannot manage him alone. It takes the two of us a couple of hours to get him to bed.

If nothing works, it is not your fault – and your charge's poor memory will be a boon, because they will quickly forget the episode. You, however, may still feel helpless, limp and washed out. It is no fun to be sworn at, threatened or hit by someone you are caring for, especially if you used to be close to – and loved by – them.

It is better to leave them alone in mid-stream anger (unless they are wrecking the place) and go and let out your own feelings to a helpful listener. This might be a person who relates well with the aggressive person and can distract them.

If things get totally out of control, press their medical alarm button or dial the emergency services.

Other strong reactions
Extreme tears or laughter

A person with dementia who has previously scared you with their aggression may confuse you by weeping or laughing uncontrollably – at quite inappropriate moments or seemingly out of proportion to anything that has happened. This is another example of their response system's increasingly defective 'wiring'. New places, loud noises, unfamiliar people and large groups, or uncertainty about a task, may lead to weeping rather than shouting or striking out.

The usual response is called for: a long, quiet, empathetic hug, and then a distraction. It might be worth your while to make a list of immediate distractions you can call on if needed.

The involuntary grip

Sometimes the person you are caring for may shake hands with someone, and hurt them without intending to, by going on and on with an extra-strong grip. This is involuntary: your friend's muscles have contracted and do not let go.

> Colin, in hospital again with a nasty infection, was sitting by a window when Gwenda arrived. He scarcely acknowledged her but shot out his hand, grasped her wrist and pulled her towards him. 'Get me out of this place,' he growled. Gwenda felt her wrist hurt as she resisted him and he clung on powerfully.
>
> She relaxed and let her arm remain passive, while talking to him and unfolding his fingers one at a time to free herself, uncovering the inch-long slit where his grip had torn her paper-thin skin. Without comment she pulled out a large handkerchief, wrapped it round her arm and went on matter-of-factly telling him local news. It was months before she learned that the 'death grip' is common in dementia.

If a person with dementia grabs you and won't let go, try gently massaging their fingers towards their wrist, and prising them off one by one. If their hands want to grip the wrong things, give them a rolled-up facecloth or hand towel, or a small hand-exercise ball to squeeze.

Making sense of it, managing the future
Consider your role

When an aggressive outburst is over and done with, and you are able to reflect calmly, consider what may underlie your charge's aggression, and any role you may have had in this. When you have been occupied by something else and away from them, they may protest by 'playing up'. Perhaps they use violence to get your full attention, like a child who acts naughtily just to get their mother to take notice of them. You may realise in retrospect that you routinely give your charge a cuddle when they stop being violent, thus rewarding the bad behaviour. If you interact with them more often at irregular intervals (not regularly, otherwise they expect it), you may side-step the aggression.

If you frequently feel stirred up or impatient with your charge, this may be a clue that you need more help in your caring job. Be aware, too, that you may need a safe outlet for your feelings: expressing them can take pressure off for both of you. (See Chapter 12: Feelings.)

Use your journal

Write up your journal while your memory is fresh, with the dates and times of any aggressive outbursts. Let the person you are caring for see you doing it and include them by asking for their ideas. They are still their own person inside, with thoughts and intuitions. They may be a fruitful source of personal solutions.

Ask yourself these questions in relation to any one incident:
- Who was present?
- What personal interactions preceded the outburst?
- What was the person with dementia doing at the time when things erupted?
- What would they have been feeling?
- What were you, the carer, doing and feeling?
- What do you consider may have caused the upset?
- What did you do when the eruption occurred?
- How successful was this response?

When you need to consider more than one incident – a series, perhaps – consult your journal for clues and ask yourself about any patterns you can sense, such as:
- time of day (sundowning, mealtime, bedtime)
- the setting (at home, out walking, in a crowd, in a strange place)
- people present or absent (family members, different staff at day care)
- particular activities (invasion of their privacy, a new game).

Work out where the aggression is directed, whether at you, a person in uniform, strangers, or some other type of person. Warning signs can be important, too, so consider whether these are becoming evident and, if so, note them in your journal. Are they always followed by a violent act? If not, note what you did that was different in your journal so that violence is averted in future.

Look into possible medical reasons for the incidents, including inadequate or poorly fitting glasses and hearing aids. Try to find out if your charge has unidentified pain, discomfort, undiagnosed illness, depression, or side-effects from medications.

Problem-solving and prevention

Once you have identified a reason or reasons for an aggressive episode, you might like to work out a list of ways you could have responded. Apply problem-solving techniques for selecting a solution to try. (Adapt steps 4–8 in Chapter 12: Feelings, 'Problem-solving'.) Put down your craziest ideas!

Remember that generally, the best atmosphere for your charge is a simple, repetitive routine in the same environment among the same people. Ensuring this atmosphere may be a good way to avoid a sense of their feeling overwhelmed, powerless or unfairly treated.

Frequent eruptions

If aggression erupts too frequently for comfort, seek help: a medical assessment from your doctor if your charge hasn't had one fairly recently; or advice from the dementia foundation specific to the condition. If you feel you are continually in physical danger it is imperative that you report it to one of your health-care team. They should guide you to the best source of relief.

Whether or not aggressive incidents happen again, use the helpful agencies (see Useful Resources). Other people have new ideas and different experiences, and may suggest ways to avoid aggression.

Where to from here

+ Chapter 10: Wider Support and Self-care
+ Chapter 12: Feelings
+ Chapter 13: Communication
+ Chapter 14: Intimacy, Love and Sex
+ Chapter 23: Hallucinations, Delusions and Delirium

Part Six

The Later Stages

Chapter 25

Choosing Full-time Care

Hard decisions

For someone who retains even a shred of understanding, going into full-time care is one of the worst times of their life. But it may be unavoidable. Perhaps they have become too frail to stay at home.

> Lindsay's dementia began after a clot blocked his carotid artery and his brain was starved of blood. He had been a gentle, kind giant of a man, and the dementia seemed to make him just a little gentler and kinder, but then one of his knees collapsed, and his dementia worsened after the anaesthetic for the necessary surgery. Diabetes and gout added to his woes, and eventually he had to have one leg amputated below the knee. Jane could manage no longer. He needed full-time care.

A home carer can also, like Jane, come to the end of their tether. Perhaps their own health has packed up partly because of the nature of their work looking after their charge.

The eventual decision to ask for a referral for full-time care may be made by you alone, you and your charge, or both of you together with the family. However, the people who make the final decision are your doctors and someone with clinical qualifications, supported by a specialist in geriatric care. In some countries this decision may be backed up by a psychogeriatrician, who will decide what level of care and what drugs or treatment are needed. You and other close family members may disagree, but professional advice is hard to ignore.

Often people with dementia feel they were not consulted about when and where they should go into care. So it is important that, if possible, you talk things over with the person you are looking after – even if you fear a negative response.

The possibility of full-time care was brought up with one woman with dementia who said dismissively, 'I've got daughters, and they will care for me in my home.' It took many weeks of planning, and many conferences between the family and her medical team, before she grudgingly agreed to move into a safe retirement complex.

Reluctance to move

Some people with dementia, living with a carer at home, do not recognise when this is no longer possible and refuse point blank to go anywhere else. Or they may have been content to live alone, not realising how much effort their visiting family members, friends and social workers have put into looking after them, or that these carers worry constantly about fire, falls or other accidents. They become furious and indignant in response to suggestions that they need more help or 'sheltered housing'. Very seldom do they agree.

A 103-year-old matriarch refused to move into full-time care. She was looked after by her daughter, a senior citizen who was also caring for her own 90-year-old husband.

The latter's sharp brain finally found the successful strategy. In cahoots with the matron of the chosen retirement home, the daughter began taking her mother once a week to the facility's hairdressing salon, and one day simply did not collect her mother after her appointment. Instead, the staff took her to her new room. There was a bit of a kerfuffle, but the mother finally acknowledged she was beaten and became a matriarch in her new home.

Your experience may not be as extreme as this, though your charge may grumble and groan, even after the move. However, if you choose the place carefully, they will probably be as well looked after as if they were in their own home – and perhaps better in some cases. They will also form new attachments.

Investigating costs
Check your eligibility for funding

Enquire with the relevant authority about the costs of full-time care. Begin by having a needs assessment. This, combined with income and asset testing, will clarify the level of state residential care subsidy for which you are eligible. If you are not eligible, you may be entitled to a loan.

The cost of caring is often more than the financial help you receive. Check with your support organisation that you are getting all the national sickness or senior citizen benefits you are eligible for.

The next financial step

Be prepared to talk about your finances with your family, accountant or the home manager when you have chosen a place. At that point you will need to find out when accounts are sent; also when and how they can be paid. For instance, you may be able to arrange direct credits from your government pension scheme.

Check what is included in the fees. You need to know what the facility classes as 'extras'; for example, telephone use, incontinence pads, soaps and toothpaste, fruit juices, biscuits and snacks.

Given your charge is in a new living situation, you may now qualify for the single person's pension rate. It is also sensible to consider whether your current medical insurance policies will still be necessary or useful.

> After Donald died Helen carried on working. She felt the relief of 20 years of physical caring taken off her shoulders, but the struggle to pay the bills remained. When she received the account from their private health insurers, however, she realised she had been paying quite unnecessary premiums since Donald had gone into full-time care. He had had free medical care in the home and during his several trips to the local public hospital.

Check about the system for doctors' visits and medication needs. How are prescriptions supplied? Can you negotiate their costs?

When an injury is suspected after a fall, a residential facility may call in the portable X-ray company, but your permission should be sought. The state may contribute a portion of the cost.

Looking for a place

You may be looking for a rest home, a dementia unit, a hospital offering long-term care or a psychogeriatric hospital; it depends on your charge's needs. Ideally you will already have gathered relevant brochures and begun considering possible places. If you haven't, don't leave it too long. Avoid making a snap decision, and make sure you talk to:

- your organisation's support person
- doctors and specialists
- fellow support group members
- staff in the day-care facility your charge attends
- community helpers who come to your home to wash and dress your charge
- management and families of people with dementia in places you are considering.

Then go over everything with the person you are looking after, weighing up how the different places will suit, or what they lack. You may feel you are talking to yourself a lot of the time, if your charge's understanding and speech are slow, but keep them in the picture. It can be stunning to discover how much they understand without showing it.

Their usual respite care facility may seem an obvious choice, but may not be suitable. It may not have a secure unit, or the person's wandering or aggression may have developed too much. Sometimes an institution's full-time care facilities are inferior to its day-care facilities.

> Humphrey had been attending a very well-run day care for two years, and said he would like to go into the hospital associated with it when he needed full-time care. But people who had had relatives in the hospital said 'No': it had too few and poorly trained staff, tiny, inconvenient rooms, suspect sanitation, and management who didn't listen. It was amazing to find two facilities run together by the same corporate owner, with such different standards.

Sometimes the place sells itself, and you feel it's right soon after walking in the door, but make sure you still ask lots of questions of the managers.

Look for a home which is well recommended, with easy access and parking. Ideally it will have no more than 20 residents and be equipped to care for your charge's form of dementia. Make a list of questions before you go; don't be embarrassed to ask them.

It may help you to choose your facility if you put ticks and crosses beside the following suggestions and pointers.

The room
Unless your charge is bed-bound and incontinent, look for a room that:
- is single, airy, clean and homelike, not clinical
- offers enough space for armchair, chest of drawers, television and so on
- has a cork notice-board or walls, easily reached and visible from the bed, for attaching photos and family memorabilia
- has its own bathroom, with floor sloping to a drainage point, individual or shared with only one other resident
- has night-lights, telephone and television points, adequate wardrobe and storage space
- is away from high traffic areas, and has a garden view as well as easy, direct access to securely fenced areas outside, in case of wandering.

Wider resources, activities
Find out where and how patients spend their days. Are they moved to different areas for stimulation, if appropriate? Given that dementia patients feel safer with regularity, enquire whether there is a daily or weekly routine and, if so, whether this is balanced with flexibility. You may want to know if your charge will have a telephone or, if not, how easily they can get access to one. Ask, too, if alcohol is allowed.

Check if the home has:
- a large communal lounge and dining area for uncrowded socialising
- smaller sitting rooms for one-on-one visits
- good light and sunny corners inside (remember, older people need much better light than younger people)
- access to kitchen facilities where residents can make drinks and snacks

- a day-care room with regular activities that all residents can attend
- physiotherapy and occupational therapy facilities.

Other factors are whether the home you are considering owns a van and arranges outings. Does it have a garden plot where they can potter, perhaps with visitors? This could be more practical than bringing them flowers or pot plants!

> One woman picked the heads off flowers given to her and 'replanted' them on her floral carpet, while another woman used her floral bedspread to 'repot' the plants visitors had brought her. Where better to do it?

Hygiene

Look (and sniff!) for the hygiene standards. Detectable urine or faecal odours anywhere are not good. Are rubber gloves readily available for the nurses, and do they use them? Gloves should always be used when there is likely contact with any bodily fluids or substances.

What is the home's policy on showering and hygiene? If you discover later that your charge has not been showered, and feel let down, check that the staff members are not actually deferring to your charge's wishes. Sometimes they will feel just too tired or out of sorts to be bothered with getting undressed and washed. They should not be bullied or manhandled.

> Visiting Bruce at his full-time care facility one morning, Alison found him slumped in his chair with his eyes closed. 'What's happened, darling?' she said, hugging him and kissing his forehead. He groaned. Then, stumblingly, he told her how 'those big nurses' had forced him to have a shower when he didn't want one. 'They were terribly rough.' Distressed, she had a word with the head nurse, who dismissed her concerns. Her staff would never be like that – but they had been ordered to shower all patients every day.

It is a good idea to ask how incontinence is managed. Is there a bladder training programme? Only a minimal percentage of the residents should be on catheters. Find out if the home uses air mattresses or 'egg carton' foam pads, which help prevent bedsores. Bedsores are not a good sign, so be assertive; ask how many residents have them.

Food

If meals come from large-scale commercial caterers, enquire about their reputation. If food is prepared 'in house', wander into the kitchen and scan the surfaces and procedures.

Ask to see a week's menu. How appetising and nutritious are the meals? An unannounced visit at mealtime will soon tell you. Find out whether staff members will, if necessary, help residents to eat their meals and monitor intake.

How often are meals served on a tray in resident's rooms? If too often, they can feel lonely; but sometimes they will grumble about table mates in the dining room and request 'room service'!

Meeting the people

Assessing the people who work in a home is at least as important as checking the place and space. Find out what training staff receive in understanding and managing the behaviour of people with dementia. Do you see lots of fun, laughter and joking? What use will they make of your charge's life book and medical folder? (See Chapter 6: Becoming a Carer.)

The staff–patient ratio is significant. Ask, specifically, how many residents they have per caregiver. Three caregivers to 25 residents would be a good daytime ratio, and two to 25 at night-time. In a nursing home situation a registered nurse is not legally required, but having one always available for nursing home and dementia unit residents is a good sign.

Check how often the physiotherapist and occupational therapist attend, as well as viewing the room they work in. What medical service does the home provide? The number of doctors who attend, and how frequently, are important points. With complex medical problems it is better to have your own doctor, or for them to brief the home's doctors.

Assess senior staff carefully but unobtrusively. They set the tone of the place and must be caring, competent and sincere. You need to feel comfortable with them because you will have ongoing contact.

A place which does not measure up in all these areas, but where you see the residents calm and happy, and the staff relaxed, laughing and interacting with them, could be the right choice.

As you look around, another thing to check is whether residents are encouraged to do as much for themselves as possible. Again, there's a balance to achieve: care and attention must always be available, but independence (where possible) is important too.

Rights and protection

Look for a list of residents' rights, posted prominently. Are these followed? Other initiatives to promote communication and participation could include:

- a newsletter to update residents on activities, changes to the system, or names of new arrivals
- a residents' committee, whose evaluations and recommendations are noted and acted upon – people with dementia may still like to contribute.

Personal security is another consideration, so you should ask not just about the security of a locked dementia unit but about the visiting policy of any facility you are investigating: whether visitors have to sign in, and if they can come at any time.

You may appreciate being allowed to stay for meals with your charge or to sleep over, but such visitation rights need balancing with protection for all residents. This may seem fussy; but there have been cases of burglary and assault, including sexual assault, in nursing homes.

Use of restraints

Is there a non-restraint policy, or do staff members strap people into chairs and wheelchairs? In some countries, each time a person is physically restrained in a care facility, a doctor or nurse must complete a chart to circulate among the staff, so that the person is not left for longer than two consecutive hours.

Restraints may not just mean preventing someone from walking about:

> In one nursing home a tradesman saw a resident with her mouth taped shut. The temporary caregiver could not stand her constant calling out so had taken thoughtless and illegal steps to prevent it.

Medicating to manage difficult behaviour or exercise 'social control' is another form of restraint. This practice has been alarmingly widespread in care facilities with, according to one statistic, 50 per cent of homes reputed to use antipsychotic drugs regularly.

When you are choosing a facility for your charge, find out its policy on the use of sedatives, tranquillisers and hypnotic drugs. Are they used frequently, or only as a last resort?

If people are medicated to calm them down or send them to sleep, this can make the problem behaviour worse, because these chemicals work by slowing the brain down. Their many possible side-effects include: drowsiness; increased confusion and disorientation; dizziness; falls; tremor; constipation; incontinence; loss of self-motivation, self-care and daily living skills; and insomnia. (See also Chapter 15: Maintaining Health, 'Cautionary notes'.)

> A husband found his spouse zonked out and strapped into a wheelchair, sitting in wet pants and staring vacantly into space among several other patients in the same condition. He was told she had to be sedated because she had wandered off and become aggressive when brought inside.

Some doctors claim they use such drugs to reduce suffering. But the suffering is probably that of the other residents, staff, and visitors.

The best places use minimal medication, and trained and motivated staff. They aim to give each individual the best quality of life possible, and welcome any help offered. With common sense and lateral thinking, it may be possible to avoid either a physical or pharmaceutical straitjacket.

> In one dementia unit, where a patient kept getting out of his chair and causing trouble, the staff didn't use a restraint. They wondered whether he was simply bored and needed more stimulation, so they put his chair by the office, where people were coming and going all day, and the problem disappeared.

A carer's ongoing involvement

It's in the best interests of your charge for the family and/or the principal carer to continue being involved in their life at their new home, so think about how you can participate. Does the management like help from volunteers? You could offer to drive a sight-seeing or pick-up-and-drop-off van for them. When carers come in and help at weekends, during staff shortages, residents may be less anxious and agitated.

Alternatively, you could join or form a carers' support group, or even a Friends Committee for the facility itself. Dozens of community organisations (orchestras, museums, theatre companies and art galleries and the like) have such groups; there is no reason why a residential care facility shouldn't have one too.

Find out about the institution's expectations of carers: they may want you to do mending and other small jobs. What do you need to tell management if you are going away? Ask, if the person going into care is your partner, whether you can have privacy when you visit, as closeness and intimacy are so necessary for couples. You need to know, too, at what stage management will let you know if your charge falls down or becomes ill.

What is the procedure if you need to make a complaint – or if a problem arises in your resident's care? Will you be included in any staff conferences to find solutions?

> Vernon had caused many problems for the staff since he went into the home. Zoe was very aware of them and told the matron that she would like to help if she could. She was impressed – and a little intimidated – to be summoned to a meeting with three bigwigs of the home's management; but she was also impressed by the way they discussed and tried sympathetically to solve Vernon's situation with her help.

Check the facility's discharge policy. You need to know their criteria and conditions if you wish, or need, to change homes.

When the choice is made
Arranging a trial stay

It is worth negotiating for your charge to have a trial stay for a few weeks, with no legal commitments to continue. Attend residents' activity sessions at the home several times a week to get a feel for the place. In the meantime, don't sell your present home or property.

> Before my mother went as a resident to the home, I took her about three times a week for the day, to get her used to the place. She didn't want to go, and I felt mean, but the staff told me she was okay when she got there.

After taking these precautions, you and your charge should have a fairly clear overall picture of the place you choose. Hopefully, you will feel satisfied that you have planned carefully and covered everything.

Sign a contract

Ask for a clear contract which covers all the considerations of this chapter, and in which all possible extras and potential costs are set out. Any extra charges should not be incurred without your consent or that of the relevant person with Enduring Power of Attorney.

From this point, you should be able to get on with the business of loving, and leave the caring to the facility.

Where to from here

- ✦ Chapter 5: Legal and Money Matters
- ✦ Chapter 6: Becoming a Carer
- ✦ Chapter 7: Dealing with Health Professionals
- ✦ Chapter 10: Wider Support and Self-care
- ✦ Chapter 11: Independence and Safety
- ✦ Chapter 17: Entertainment
- ✦ Chapter 26: Moving into Full-time Care
- ✦ Chapter 27: Final Days

Chapter 26

Moving into Full-time Care

The move itself

The best time to take your charge and their possessions to their room in the new home is when they are at their best. This will usually be in the morning. Try to involve them in furnishing it like their old home, with familiar touches: photo albums, flower vases, their own duvet or bedding and pillows, a favourite armchair – and anything familiar which won't clutter the room but will give them a sense of belonging.

You could decorate the walls with personal photos, familiar pictures, grandchildren's drawings or family memorabilia, while talking about the memories these evoke. Perhaps install a handy night-light and hang their name and/or photo on their door, as it will help them identify their room in this strange new place.

It is important to be sensitive, however, to their wishes. They may not be ready to accept this transformation.

> Some people refuse to have their own stuff in their room. One woman said it was not her home and never would be, so did not want anything personal there at all.

The first day

The first day in a rest home is very important. An uncluttered, uncrowded atmosphere with recognisable routines was best in your charge's familiar home of many years, so it is even more necessary in this strange new place. One carer recommends that you take the first day off work if possible, and plan to spend the entire day settling them in, as it can be an overwhelming experience.

> At one very good and welcoming place, the first day was marred by there being far too many people in my mother's room – other residents popping in to welcome her, a carpenter finishing off last-minute details, nurses introducing themselves – all well-meaning but overwhelming.

At another institution the experience was much worse:

> My mother was left unattended in the waiting room while my husband and I had to discuss treatments, the possible use of restraints and cremation/burial options, all with Mum wandering in and out of the room. It was distressing enough for us. It must have been terrifying for her.

Be there for their first meal or two, walk around the place with them (with their walker or wheelchair if they can't walk), sit and reminisce about the past. Perhaps you can lend other furnishings from their old home to this new place, so that they feel a sense of familiarity as they move around?

> One daughter introduced her mother to her new room, arranged a vase of flowers there with her, then took her home to stay the night. The transition from a home of 40 years to a rest home seemed too big to do in one day. This worked well. Another carer did the same, but her person with dementia refused to go back the next day!

Some homes ask that you don't take the new resident out for at least two to three weeks.

Clothing in hospital

Fewer clothes are needed in full-time care than at home, and those you take should be able to go through a hot wash and clothes dryer. Ensure all clothing is named, but avoid iron-on labels; they don't last long. The home may suggest a place which makes woven labels and may have a sewing service. Perhaps family or friends could help you sew them on.

Laundry goes missing all the time, despite the staff's best efforts; but it may be other patients who help themselves to your resident's clothes, or your charge who is wearing something you've never seen before.

Sometimes a cross-dresser streak comes out:
> Gareth often went into women's rooms and attired himself with obvious delight in their frocks, jackets, scarves and gloves. He never stripped right down and put on their bras and panties, though.

It is so common for clothing to go missing or unfamiliar items to appear that you may as well accept it. If your charge notices and is upset, the solution may be to do all their laundry yourself. Sometimes there can be an argument or even a physical fight over garments.

> The first time the rest home phones to tell you about such an incident you are horrified. It's as if the school principal were to ring and tell you that your child had been caught stealing or fighting. Then you realise that they are not criticising or expecting you to cringe and apologise for your resident. They are just keeping you in the loop (or possibly covering their own backs in case the situation escalates). All you need to do is say warmly, 'Thanks for letting me know.'

Your role changes

Caregiving does not stop when your charge goes into long-term care: it changes. Your role shifts from being the full-time carer to being an active advocate for their needs. As your charge may not be able to assert themselves, this is crucial.

Keep a close eye on the home's routine and its staff. For instance, you will probably want to make sure staff are sensitive to your charge's comfort level, given the inability of many people with dementia to take off or put on extra layers of clothing.

It is helpful to be aware that the way of doing things in the full-time care facility may be different from your way, so be slow to criticise. Retirement homes have usually worked out the most efficient ways of working with large numbers of fragile people.

Getting to know each other
Meet the staff

All the workers at the home are involved in the caring – even the gardeners – so it is worthwhile learning their names. You might like to think about staff members' backgrounds, their languages and attitudes – even to find out the cultural significance of words and gestures used by staff from other countries.

> Trudi's mother was in full-time care and had not spoken for many months, but one day, in Trudi's presence, her mother broke her silence – and angrily: 'That man called me darling and asked me to sit on his knee!' she blurted out, pointing at one of the dark-skinned nursing staff.
>
> The man himself was disarmingly friendly and open when Trudi approached him. 'Yes, yes, I said that. Back home that's how we treat the old luvvies. They need warmth and affection and cuddles, so we give it to them.'
>
> 'Well, in our country that's not what our oldies expect or need from strangers,' Trudi replied. Later, though, she felt she had been a bit stuffy.

Offer insights into your charge

As a home-based carer you may have much to offer people who look after your charge in the place you have chosen. One thing is to help the carers learn something about your charge's background. Make a point of showing your charge's life book to staff, so they will get some insights into the person and discover subjects to chat about. This can defuse agitation and any possible aggression: it is beneficial for all concerned.

> One man with dementia lived on his own and liked to get up early to do some gardening before breakfast. His family, who kept a regular eye on him, thought he would be safer in care while they travelled – with dire consequences. The facility where they took him tried to make him fit in to their timetable, and this quiet man became very aggressive and violent when they tried to restrict his usual habits. The family hadn't created a life book to leave with him.
>
> ◆
>
> Staff in another place noticed that a new resident was aimless, unhappy and didn't join in activities. Her life book told them she had been a teacher, so they tried putting chalk, a blackboard and

duster in her room. She fiddled about with them often and seemed much more content.

You may like to consider placing a visitors' book in the room, for people to record when they call in. This can be a talking point afterwards, with staff reassuring your charge that they are not forgotten. The rest home workers may also appreciate being told whether your charge prefers rest and quiet – away from noisy television or radio or patients with annoying habits – or a more sociable atmosphere.

Spending time with your charge

Try to be at their new home a lot at first. A very small number of carers stay all day, every day, doing things with their charge and listening. This gives the people they stay with a message that they are worthy of attention and respect, despite their dementia, and the carer is more likely to be remembered.

You may choose to be there full time yourself, as you work out the best and easiest ways to get your charge through their first days. Such attendance is very rare, however, and very rarely possible, though it may seem ideal.

In most places, if you are there all the time, you will be welcomed as almost one of the staff. In others, the staff may seem wary that you are spying on them.

Frequency, regularity

Often the secret objective of visiting is to make the visitor feel good. You don't have to visit every day. You could keep tabs on who else calls in and, perhaps, make an informal timetable including them. This will give you opportunities to attend special events, or simply have a day off. Carers need variety and other people to mix with.

> One daughter, who visited her mother regularly, intentionally didn't mention that she was going to Spain for a month. On her return, her mother seemed delighted to see her. She didn't even say, 'Where have you been? You haven't been to see me for ages!', which she usually snapped when her daughter left her for 10 minutes on a normal visit. The daughter felt quite hurt!

When you visit, it is good to have a range of peaceful and familiar activities to choose from, such as:
- sorting clothes in the bedroom
- throwing bread to birds
- singing together inside
- eating together
- joining other residents for entertainment in the lounge.

The comfort of routine, for the person with dementia, makes it best to do the same things in the same place each time – for instance, identifying a particular seat in the garden and making the short trip to that favourite place. (Variety, though more stimulating for you, can confuse them after a certain stage.)

Visit at irregular times, however. Dementia does not mean people affected cannot read the time.

> One woman was determined to be the perfect wife when her husband went into permanent care. She told him she would come in every day about 2 pm. And so she did, until the first time she was unavoidably delayed for an hour or so.
>
> When she arrived, hot and bothered, he was sitting in his chair absolutely furious. 'Where have you been!' he shouted. 'Look at the clock – ten past three! I've been waiting all this time. It's not good enough. Here I am, stuck in this place, and you can't even be considerate enough.' He ranted for ages. 'Perfection' had not paid off.

What to take when visiting

Pets, especially familiar ones, are popular visitors. Dogs are not judgemental about dementia, and will tail-wag and slobber in their usual doggy way. Other patients can also enjoy animals and find their visits therapeutic.

If you are a parent, you could take your baby with you and, perhaps, ask the person you are visiting if they would like to hold the child. They may love that and do so comfortably if they have been a parent themselves. If they have not, find out tactfully if they are used to holding babies.

A simple bunch of flowers, even a single bloom, can be a lovely gift, especially if it's from their former garden. Arranging flowers gives you something in the present to talk about, avoiding 'What have you been doing/had for lunch?', which can be confusing because it is in the recent past.

Visiting tips

- ✦ Try to keep questions out of your conversation.
- ✦ If the person you are visiting seems uneasy with the noise and activity, find a quieter spot to sit in.
- ✦ Holding hands or touching somehow helps interaction.

Taking people with dementia out

If you take someone out for a trip or a treat, it is considerate to go back with them to their room when you bring them home. Most people with dementia benefit from this. Even after they have been in full-time care for ages, they 'forget' the home while they are out, and it helps to have you there while they settle back.

When dementia is well advanced, nursing home staff sometimes say not to take the person out at all, because they can become disoriented and distressed while out or on their return.

> As a treat we arranged to take Granny, confused and in a nursing home, to visit her very elderly mother – our great-granny – out in the country. We left Granny in the car when we stopped to buy something, and found her standing in the middle of the road amidst heavy traffic when we came back. She was trying to flag down a lift back to the nursing home. 'Matron wouldn't like me to be out like this,' she explained.
>
> When we eventually arrived at our great-granny's place, Granny soon disappeared from the living room and we found her sitting primly on her bed, saying again, 'Matron wouldn't approve,' and asking where were the street lights and trees she usually saw outside her nursing-home window.

When visiting is not easy

If you feel reluctant to visit, you could try modelling yourself on someone who seems to cope well, and push yourself along. You may feel really satisfied afterwards, and allow yourself a pat on the back.

If you are not well received when you go reluctantly, perhaps the person you are visiting reads you well. Perhaps you give negative messages – a stiff unsmiling attitude, frowns or head shakes? Leave and go more happily another time.

If your charge has been horrible and aggressive, and you are feeling hurt and unforgiving in return, it is a good idea to stay away for a period to collect yourself. They may not be aware of the time gap and, usually, the hiatus allows you to understand that they are not actually responsible for their behaviour. You may not be so upset next time.

When the person concerned is not a 'loved one'

Most literature on dementia speaks about dealing with 'your loved one'. Let's face it, often the person you have been caring for is not a 'loved one'. They can be 'put up with' – often grudgingly – and once they are in permanent care, you feel 'At last! Thanks be.' You never want to see them again, and do not want to keep in touch.

There are ways to fulfil any obligations you may still feel:
- keep them supplied with everyday necessities
- give financial support, or provide other practical help, to their new home.

Let the home's manager know your true feelings; they are not uncommon. The manager should understand, and you may feel better if you get 'stuff' off your chest.

Leave the home your contact details. It may help them later to have someone to talk to who has known your charge for a while, who can be approached for information and permission for interventions.

Don't believe that you have to like someone to love them. Mother Teresa didn't know the thousands of people she looked after. She didn't know whether she liked or disliked them; she simply cared for them with love.

Should you employ a helper?

Occasionally it may be wise to employ a helper or minder when your charge goes into full-time care. A person with dementia may be very scared when they are in new surroundings and darkness sets in.

> Zita was having her third move in as many months, so her family found a qualified nurse to be a daily helper with her in her new home. Sanji was wonderful. She saw that Zita was smartly dressed, took her on outings and to the hairdresser, and the move went remarkably smoothly.
>
> Unfortunately the new home protested that they were responsible if anything happened to Zita while she was out of their environs, and Sanji felt she would be wasted just filling in time in the home – and resigned.

You may be able to afford to employ your own carers; but, if your budget is strained, explore the health department helpers – they can be soundly experienced and empathetic – or ask church or local volunteer groups.

Feelings and reactions
Your feelings

Your feelings may have been challenging when you were the primary carer, but your charge's move to a home or hospital can produce new and strong emotions.

> Edgar had often been very upset when his wife railed at him during her illness, and so had developed a hard shell around himself. It had been his only way to cope. Edgar reported that he felt solitary, alone and in limbo while he was caring for her, because there was no one else around he could talk to.
>
> When she was taken to hospital his feelings overcame him: he felt he hadn't been affectionate enough – had been too hard. He felt terribly guilty. Finding himself alone in their empty home after the years of looking after her, he asked himself 'What do I do now?'

Relief – that you no longer have to cope with everything – is understandable, though difficult to admit. If the one you have been looking after is a spouse, sibling or parent with whom you have never got on well, and you have looked after them from a great sense of duty, you don't have to feel guilty at feeling relieved.

Guilt can still emerge at not having done enough to show affection (as in the story above), or at some other 'failure' that you blame yourself for.

Related feelings can include shame at not being able to continue, when others do; and worry that people will think you hard-hearted.

Loneliness is common, too, after being so over-occupied for years.

After Leah had settled her mother into her long-term care home, the home's manager showed her out, saying she'd 'done her bit'. But Leah was despondent and wasn't ready to go home to an empty house. What she really needed was a bit of sympathy from the manager.

You may feel a sense of loss, from coping with a 'living death' and because the person you know is no longer 'there'. Sadness, too, is a core emotion: this may be about losing your charge, or all the things you couldn't do during the time you spent caring.

Things can seem strange and unreal for a while, even frightening. 'Am I going mad?' you may wonder. Alternatively you may feel anxious, wondering how your charge will manage in their new setting. Will they be well looked after? Might they reject you for 'doing this' to them?

Other natural reactions are: anger that others didn't help more when it was needed, so that your charge could have stayed at home longer; fear that one day this might happen to you; or helplessness – at not still being in control, after battling against all the odds for so long.

It's fair to say you may face a whole smorgasbord of unresolved emotions, especially if you lost control when a crisis intervened and decisions about the future of your charge were taken out of your hands.

Whatever has led up to the move, you can expect:

✦ to find it hard to sleep, especially with no one beside you, no one to put your arms around
✦ days to seem long and empty
✦ to feel that you have failed.

My profound physical exhaustion has eased, and in its place I have feelings of desolation and inadequacy and an ever-present financial worry which, after our efforts to provide for an independent old age, I did not expect. Not least, there is also the daily trauma of leaving him.

You may also be surprised to find physical changes; that you lose muscle tone because you are no longer lifting and meeting other daily demands of caring.

Ten tips for getting through it

1. Talk with your support group, with others who've been through it.
2. In bed at night, try putting your arm round a pillow. If you no longer have your constant companion, this may help a little.
3. Ask your friends in for meals.
4. Visit a returned services' club or service organisation to eat out or socialise.
5. Get a job.
6. Take up long-neglected hobbies and other interests.
7. Start studying through U3A (an international network of retired people who want to learn), community colleges, extramural university courses.
8. Spoil yourself. If you have spare time, spend it on grooming and dressing up when going out.
9. See all the talked-about films and plays or go to rock concerts, the speedway, exhibitions.
10. Take up regular, ongoing exercise: swimming, cycling or walking (longer distances each week); or horse riding; golf; tennis; dancing; going to a gym; aerobics; tai chi; health and fitness classes; yoga.

Your charge's reactions

In the first few weeks your charge may be discontented and grieving; but later they become comfortably 'institutionalised', as they settle into the ways of the home.

> One new resident caused a few laughs by saying the pastures here
> must be good because all the nurses are nice and fat.

New people in their life will provide care and affection. Don't be too upset if, over time, they show attachment to a particular member of staff or another patient. It often happens. People want someone to love.

Later, when you visit, you may find them clean and content – or morose, complaining or argumentative. Are these latter behaviours unlike them? If you feel uneasy, and their unhappiness is out of character, find out tactfully about their daily behaviour, interactions with staff and so on. Speak with the management. Their reactions may show something which needs investigation.

New challenges
When they don't speak
Staying away may feel easier if your charge has lost the power of speech, but continue to be in regular contact. Talk to them, even though they don't reply. (See Chapter 13: Communication, 'When the person no longer speaks'.)

Create a special occasion sometimes. Bring in a drink and nibbles and play dominoes or a game that doesn't need much talk. Have lots of physical touching if they like it: hugs, arms round shoulders, brushing hair, rubbing cream into their hands and feet. (They may like to rub cream into yours, too.)

Organise your 'keeping in touch' so that you will last the distance. There may be years ahead of you.

Weight loss
Weight loss and even malnutrition often occur in people with moderate or severe dementia in nursing homes. There can be several reasons, usually nothing to do with small helpings:
- Your charge may have lost the ability to chew or swallow.
- Perhaps they can't handle cutlery to get food to their mouth, don't know that food is to be eaten, or can't concentrate on finishing their meal.
- Deteriorating eyesight may mean they can't see food on the edge of their plate.

If perception and/or movement are reduced in any of these ways, you may need to make sure they have staff helping them to eat at mealtimes.

Other possibilities are that they have toothache, or that their tastes have changed from sweet food to savoury (or vice versa) and the cook doesn't know. These problems, too, can be overcome; it's a matter of identifying them.

The tasty, protein-energy oral supplements now available in several flavours have helped nursing-home residents increase their weight. Ask your doctor to prescribe one. They are usually available through the health system once prescribed. (See Chapter 19: Eating and Drinking, 'Encourage a reluctant eater'.)

Is abuse mentioned?

The person you have put into full-time care may complain about abuse from the staff, sexual or otherwise. This is difficult to assess, unless you see it happening.

> One carer arrived to find his newly admitted wife with dementia being forced into her nightgown, despite her vocal protests, by staff with no training in handling people in her condition.

The behaviour of the person with dementia may lead to staff having to use physical strength to accomplish tasks like showering or toileting. Or there may be people on the staff who do, indeed, take advantage of their charges. Keep the administration informed with non-blaming, sensitive communication using 'I' messages (see Chapter 12: Feelings, 'Deal positively with your feelings') so that they become aware of possible problems and observe carefully. They cannot do this if they are not told.

> William was sitting disconsolately in his room when June arrived. His face was bruised, and he showed her marks on his body as well. 'What happened?' she asked in horror.
>
> 'They chased me last night and I couldn't get away. I fell down between a table and chair and they left me,' William murmured hoarsely.
>
> Why would they chase him? June wondered. She made discreet enquiries and was told that William had a habit of wandering during the night hours and disturbing other residents. What a difficult situation, she realised, and was not surprised when that home informed her later that they could no longer accommodate William.

Staff at the residential dementia facility you and your charge have selected should be trained to cope competently in all spheres of care. The residents' basic needs are:

- ✦ to be treated as individuals
- ✦ to have something to do each day
- ✦ to feel comfortable in – and attached to – the place in which they are living.

What a hope, though, if ward staff are among the lowest paid in the work force and receive very little training. Annual staff turnover in many homes is high, which means there is little realistic hope of residents forming close bonds with staff, or of having these basic needs met.

Possible frictions

Staff at some nursing homes may dress and undress patients roughly, speak in a demeaning way (for example, 'Now it's time we had a shower'), be selective in how they allow carers to be involved, and discourage questions from family members.

As a carer you can feel both central yet marginalised and excluded ('my husband' is 'your resident'). You may give them information yet, although you need to find things out, feel that information is withheld from you. Being sufficiently assertive is difficult: you don't want to rock the boat!

You may recognise staff knowledge, but feel your own experience is ignored. What's more, you may acknowledge pressure on staff, but see staff members 'standing around'. No wonder carers sometimes come away from visits frustrated and resentful.

> On telling the matron about her mother's complaints that she wanted to come home, a daughter was assured that the woman 'seems very content where she is and is usually in good spirits'.
>
> When the daughter insisted that she would take her mum home, the matron described various mishaps which could happen there, implying that the mother was much safer where she was. The daughter, as a result, felt pushed away and not listened to.

Many residents say they want to go home. This is seldom possible. Perhaps the matron in the story above was being realistic about the risks of going back to an ordinary family home; or perhaps she wanted to keep a fee-paying resident. Carers can initially find staff proprietorial, too, as this husband discovered:

> When Anna first went into care I thought the staff would be cross with me for changing her top and adding to the washing. Once I rang the bell because she needed to go to the toilet, but they were so slow to respond I took her myself. Then they told me off for not waiting and I was really annoyed. I've looked after Anna for years and they had no right to bully me.

Do they need to move again?

Unless the person with dementia is in the care facility because of a court order, you may shift them at any time and for any reason, giving, of course, appropriate notice to the home's management. (Refer to their policy you obtained before signing your contract.)

The reason for relocation is not always dissatisfaction. It may be that you or other regular visitors have moved to another town. However, a change should not be carried out lightly, since people with dementia find shifting stressful.

Before selecting the next home, ask for a reassessment of their condition by an appropriate geriatrician or doctor. They may be deteriorating; they may need a higher grade of nursing care and security than previously. Be there yourself for this review.

The facility should not arrange a reassessment without your consent. If they find they can no longer cope with your resident's condition, they should contact you or next-of-kin for permission to reassess.

Hospital care

If the person you have been caring for is in a nursing home with a hospital attached, be aware that, if they ever need hospital care, there may not be a bed there for them immediately. Most hospitals are run as separate economic units and aim at full occupancy.

> Gladys fell ill after being in a rest home for some time and needed hospital care. Unfortunately the rest home didn't have a hospital bed available in their facility. Her family had to decide whether to move Gladys to another private home where a hospital bed was immediately available, or to the public hospital.

Illness in hospital

Fevers and infections worsen dementia and hallucinations, and you can expect your charge to deteriorate if they are hospitalised, especially if they have an anaesthetic for an operation.

Frequently, an illness other than dementia will hasten their end, and some research suggests that palliative care for people with dementia may not be first-class during this period. Because the patient can't tell people that they are in pain, and doesn't ask for relief, painkillers are not regularly administered. You, the carer, may find yourself playing another role – guardian of pain control.

A sense of grief

Grief does not wait for death, and you may feel guilty that you are grieving while the person you have been caring for is still alive. They are not going to improve. You will both experience continual loss, and loss brings grief. Find simple books to read about what is ahead, or talk with others who have been through it.

Find your good listener, and unburden yourself regularly and thoroughly. For most people, feelings of grief become bearable if they are listened to and accepted.

Grief is an entirely natural feeling and an ongoing, cyclic experience like the ebb and flow of tides: you sink back to previous stages even while you're moving on to the next. Try to be ready.

Where to from here

- Chapter 5: Legal and Money Matters
- Chapter 7: Dealing with Health Professionals
- Chapter 11: Independence and Safety
- Chapter 12: Feelings
- Chapter 13: Communication
- Chapter 14: Intimacy, Love and Sex, especially 'In a hospital setting: intimacy with your partner'
- Chapter 17: Entertainment
- Chapter 25: Choosing Full-time Care
- Chapter 27: Final Days

Chapter 27

Final Days

Coping with final days

Dementia can cause death, but many people with dementia will die from other causes: strokes, cancer, heart attacks and so on. You may see the inevitable approaching, as your charge becomes frailer. Some people make realistic preparations. Others are taken by surprise. Still others may find intuition takes over.

> When Bill developed pneumonia after weeks of being mostly unconscious, Phyllis got in touch with their son who was away on business. 'Tell Dad to hang on for me,' he said. 'I'll be home as quickly as I can.' Phyllis gave the message to her comatose husband, but as she watched Bill struggle, fighting for every breath, she took his hand and said, 'Don't feel you've got to wait, darling. Just let go. You've been a wonderful husband to me and father to him. I love you so, but don't suffer any more.' He didn't return her hand squeeze, but his breathing eased and he died two hours later.

Allowing death and extending life

It is hard to know whether, at that stage, the person themselves has decided to let go and to die. Sometimes, however, a person with dementia does make that final decision, whether by refusing food or more actively taking their own life. It can be incredible to realise that they can still take things into their own hands, despite their seemingly overpowering dementia, like the managing director mentioned in the Introduction.

For some luckless carers, final days go on and on. It is hard to know what's best to do.

> Ralph was in long-term hospital care with advanced dementia, but he also had very painful arthritis and swallowing difficulties. His wife, Dianne, spent months assenting to different treatments until, eventually, his doctors suggested that a PEG (Percutaneous Endoscopic Gastronomy tube, which puts liquidised foods directly into the stomach) would side-step the swallowing problem. She was going to grasp at this last hope until she suddenly realised how this would just extend his life of nil quality and dreadful exhaustion. She said no and finally let nature take its course.

Sometimes a carer has to fight the doctors' desire to save a life that is clearly ending.

> Drew was going steadily downhill: his blood pressure was way down and renal failure had set in. His wife, Virginia, accepting he was dying, saw a 'Code Blue' on his hospital chart and asked what it meant. 'It means RESUSCITATE,' said the charge nurse. 'But he's got a living will,' Virginia stormed. 'That's it, then,' the nurse said. 'We'll put that on his sheet. We'll let him go.'
>
> Nevertheless the doctors on duty insisted on beginning emergency procedures, despite Virginia's protests. She rushed out and phoned the specialist, who appeared quickly and ordered the doctors to honour Drew's wishes. But five days later, after he had a massive stroke, Virginia again had to keep the doctors at bay during the short time before he died.

The necessary arrangements
Funeral planning

It can be sensible – and a bonding experience – to discuss funeral arrangements with your charge well before death. After all, how can you be sure who is going to die first? Having a pre-paid funeral arranged is an excellent idea. A funeral file can also be of great use to you or your family when the time comes, provided it is up to date and people know where to find it.

Edgar and Rosie had attended a 'Grief, Death and Dying' seminar in their fifties and, as a result, had made up separate funeral files. But, when Edgar died in his seventies, his file was out of date: they had moved to another suburb and church, his nominated minister had retired, and one or two of his chosen pallbearers had died before him. His favourite hymns and readings were still available, though!

Finances and legal loose ends

Funeral wishes are not the only information you may need to review before the death of the person you have been caring for. Much like ministers and pallbearers, trustees and executors are apt to move on.

After Theo's death, Verna found her coping abilities, built up during his long period with dementia, frustrated because his trustees had moved out of the area without telling her. One now lived on the other side of the world.

If you are the partner of the person with dementia, there are dozens of things to see to after their death. This is one reason why it is good to have done as much as you could at an earlier stage, while they were not only alive but also still able to put their signature to legal documents.

Phyllis felt prepared to cope with Dennis's death – after all, she had had years to get ready. What she was not prepared for was the stubbornness of some company managers as she went about changing the names on their accounts. One manager wouldn't consider cooperating until she provided her marriage certificate.

Sometimes, bureaucracy and its requirements mean the world appears to be solidly against you.

Sylvia felt state agencies had treated her like a fraudster when she approached them for a hospital benefit. They growled she had plenty of savings in her bank account, and she fled without pursuing her claim. After Phillip's death, however, she plucked up courage to go back and apply for a widow's pension.

Challenged to prove her circumstances were much reduced, she returned with bank statements showing that 'all that money in the bank' had been used up paying for Phillip's funeral expenses, leaving her with only $1000 in the world. She had proved her eligibility, but still had to wait weeks for the first payment.

Organ donation

Most funeral homes have booklets giving information about grief and what you need to see to, both before a funeral and afterwards; but they do not mention donating organs. That is for the family to arrange with the organisation that will eventually receive the organs.

The deceased person's organs, even very elderly ones, may be valuable to someone. Brain banks greatly value donated brains from people with dementia, although not every brain is accepted. Arrangements need to be made early and activated immediately after death, but this can be difficult for the grieving family.

> Rod cared for Lucy lovingly during the years of her Lewy body dementia and, when she died, he arranged the funeral and cremation with calm efficiency. It was only as he left the crematorium after the service that he realised he had not arranged for her brain to go to the brain bank. They had talked about this in the early days of her illness, but had not written anything down. His omission weighed heavily on him.

Dealing with how you feel

Your prior planning, and adrenalin, can carry you through the final arrangements, the funeral and the months afterwards. Be aware, though, that sudden down times will come.

> Although Theresa had arranged for Frank's brain to be donated, she found it one of the hardest aspects of his death to cope with. His brain was needed as soon as possible after death, and she just didn't want him to be taken away for its removal.

Grief

Just when you think that you are coping marvellously ('Oh, I think I'm almost over the worst'), grief hits you; and it can keep on undermining you in cycles. The busyness of life after a death has its benefits. It gives you definite tasks to concentrate on, when all you may want to do is lie down and howl.

Whatever you're feeling is what you're supposed to be feeling. Don't apologise: just as death is a natural part of life, tears are natural too. Feeling desolate is natural. Grief can be quite overwhelming – an exhausting ride; but it is an absolutely natural process and you fight expressing it at your peril. Countless people cope with it sadly but successfully every day.

The stages are the same in any grief process, from losing a pet or your job, to being sued for libel or having your whole family killed. Two years seems to be the minimum time for active grieving, although some grieve for much longer.

Time does heal (though when you are in the depths of grief, that saying is hard to accept). But no one has ever said that you eventually forget. The memory of the person who has died remains with you always; but the sharp, hurtful edges of that memory become soft pangs, rounded and treasured. We would rarely trade the experience of having and losing a loved one with never having had them at all.

Relief

If you have cared for the person with dementia for a long time, you may feel guilty because you feel relieved when they die, both for their sake and your own. You don't feel the sadness that people express sympathy for. You may feel like a hypocrite; but relief is just as natural a feeling as grief.

You probably passed through the grieving stages while you did your intensive and very practical caring. Remember those days when tears trickled down your cheeks as you drove alone in your car? Or when you walked the streets in anguish? Or when people commiserated with you? Or told you what a great job you were doing?

If the person who died is someone you found hard to be with, even before their dementia, you have even more reason to feel relieved. It is good to accept this mixture of emotions, if they are what you feel:

> Marjorie had been married to Jake for more than 60 years when he died after years of dementia and only a short illness. He had always been a difficult husband – a great bully, in fact. Ida called in to see

Marjorie a year later. 'Oh, how lovely of you to remember,' Marjorie said. 'Come in and have a drink to commemorate him.' She poured out two glasses of sherry and raised hers in a toast: 'Here's to Jake. I did hate him so, but I do miss him!'

Extreme tiredness

You may need an enormous amount of catch-up sleep if you have been a full-time carer for a long time. Perhaps you want to sleep all the time.

> Toby was constantly on the run in the seven years he looked after Ailsa. He would get her into bed every night at about 8 pm, then see to bills, phone friends, read, or watch television – things he couldn't do during the day. He went to bed late, though he knew he would be up during the night. He also knew he was desperately tired.
>
> For about a month after Ailsa's death, Toby couldn't keep his eyes open much after 7.30 pm, and he slept solidly for 11, 12 or 13 hours. Then, gradually, he could last until 7.45, then 8, then 8.15 pm until, three or four months later, he was no longer tired.

For some former carers, sleep won't come:

> Samantha had not slept well for years, even before Ron developed progressive supranuclear palsy (PSP). After he died she felt exhausted, but still did not sleep well. Whatever time she went to bed, she would wake after only a few hours of sleep. She would get up, make herself a drink and a snack and get back into bed, or into Ron's recliner chair, with a book.

One bereaved partner reported not tiredness but unexpected sexual desires.

> For years, sex between Rita and Wayne, her husband with Parkinson's dementia, was mutually difficult and frustrating. She was relieved when they changed to twin beds, although she missed his physical contact and sometimes slipped into his bed to hold him. Rita looked on her sex life as over, but quite soon after Wayne died, she was amazed that, in her seventies, she felt strong sexual urges return.

Finding support
Accept invitations

It's a good idea to accept every invitation to go out. If you say no, people may stop asking you. When with others, however, take care that you don't dominate the conversation, as you respond to people's kind enquiries. Consider warning your host that you may slip away early: either you need your sleep, or you just feel that you want to be at home.

Join new networks

Some former carers have no friends or support network around them. Maybe you have migrated recently, or your family has moved away because of work commitments, or you have no children, or you have never kept up with friends because you and the person you cared for were such a close unit. You may even not know your neighbours.

> After Kevin was diagnosed with dementia he and his wife, Rose, who were childless, started planning for their uncertain future. They moved from their large old home across the city to a small house to be near Rose's widowed sister. It was a mutually comfortable arrangement. But when Kevin died soon afterwards, things changed. The sister linked up with another partner who came to live with her and who wanted 'just the two of us'. As Rose didn't drive, she found herself stranded on her own in a strange neighbourhood.

If this is you, you now have to find your own supports. Think about joining a local church if you don't belong to one. Church people are used to people making contact in this way; it is part of what they are there for. You may find kindness and a supportive community. Alternatively, join a local club (bridge, tennis, golf, embroidery, croquet, photography), enquire at a local community support group or look in your local newspaper for activities which could give you interest, company and purpose.

Become a volunteer in the dozens of organisations which can make good use of extra hands (the art gallery, Red Cross, disabled people's groups). Look around for requests for volunteers: you can't lose if you offer your services.

For as much mental stimulation as you want, enrol in community courses in anything and everything at the local high school, or join a computer training group for seniors.

Counselling

You may always miss the person you have been caring for, but books on handling grief may help. Community groups or your doctor may have a list of grief counsellors: some are free; others charge a fee. Alternatively, find a counsellor through word of mouth. High qualifications are no guide to effective, empathetic help.

A therapist or counsellor can start you on the next part of your life as the unique individual you are; so make a series of appointments with such a person, especially if you feel that grief is lasting too long. You can emerge stronger and with more understanding.

If, after a first appointment, the chemistry between you is not right, you are best to explain and ask to see another counsellor. These therapists understand that you must feel comfortable.

Family difficulties

If family squabbles and tensions are complicating matters, a counsellor may give you the feeling of support you need. Such tensions can be just too much for you on top of everything else.

> Frank's family had been critical of his second wife, Theresa, though she tended him loyally without their help after he developed dementia. It was worse after he died. They demanded Frank's personal belongings and rights to all his money and gave her no sympathy or support. She began to cope only after seeing a counsellor.

A counsellor may arrange for you and the family members concerned to meet. Counsellors are skilled at fostering understanding between parties, but don't expect them to give advice: a good counsellor aims to help everyone at the meeting create their own blended solution. Solutions emerge if we believe in ourselves (we may need help with this), receive guidelines and are willing to work positively. The counsellor only asks the right questions of everyone and, perhaps, suggests options where they see gaps.

Reviewing, and moving on

Memories of your years as a carer may keep running through your mind. Did you do it right? You may feel remorse, because you remember times when you lost control, and other times when you feel you could have done better. You may feel regret that no one but you will ever know the minutiae of the illness: no one else will ever know the stresses and strains, the messes and stains you had to cope with, or the pride and satisfaction you felt at times.

Express your uncertain feelings to a friend – anything out in the open seems less dreadful – but balance it by congratulating yourself for the tremendous efforts you made and all the things you did so overwhelmingly right.

You may go through a period of intense grief and poignant admiration for what the person you cared for went through so uncomplainingly; or you may look back with a completely opposite view, wishing they had not gone to pieces after the diagnosis and left you to carry the whole burden.

They may have made your life a misery with their constant complaints and thick-skinned ingratitude, and you may simmer with exaggerated animosity, long suppressed, for the extended time that you 'wasted' looking after them. Then you may feel wicked for having those feelings!

Feelings, however, are the honest instincts we are born with. If you pulsate with animosity, look at it and look under it. Maybe you have good reason. This person forced you to spend more of your life on them than was fair! Perhaps it was your choice, or your animosity is really aimed at other family members who didn't take much responsibility off your shoulders. Honest acknowledgement of your feelings may clarify them, and your position too.

Although the person you cared for no longer suffers, your suffering may continue. Be ready for the down-cycles of grief to return again and again, but don't have a bad conscience when you have spells of happiness and forgetting. These will occur more frequently.

With the demands of the past over, you can pick up the things you put aside while you were a carer, and discover the new demands and opportunities of the future. There is another stage ahead, a new page on which you can plan your own priorities, cherish your own wishes and start again. Life will go on.

Where to from here
✦ Chapter 5: Legal and Money Matters
✦ Chapter 7: Dealing with Health Professionals
✦ Chapter 10: Wider Support and Self-care
✦ Chapter 12: Feelings

Useful Resources

Websites
Age Concern New Zealand: www.ageconcern.org.nz
Aged Care Australia: www.agedcareaustralia.gov.au
Alzheimer Society Canada: www.alzheimer.ca
Alzheimer Society of Ireland: www.alzheimer.ie
Alzheimer's Association (US): www.alz.org
Alzheimer's Australia: www.fightdementia.org.au
Alzheimers New Zealand: www.alzheimers.org.nz
   (also: www. wecanhelp.org.nz)
Alzheimer's Society, UK: www.alzheimers.org.uk
Alzheimer's South Africa: www.alzheimers.org.za
American Parkinson's Disease Association (APDA):
   www.apdaparkinson.org
Citizens Advice Bureau: www.cab.org.nz
Dementia Advocacy and Support Network International:
   www.dasninternational.org
Dementia Care Central (US): www.dementiacarecentral.com
Dementia UK: www.dementiauk.org
Dementia Web (UK): www.dementiaweb.org.uk/index.php
Family Services (NZ): www.familyservices.govt.nz/directory
Fisher Centre for Alzheimer's Research Foundation (US): www.alzinfo.org
GrownUps: www.grownups.co.nz
Hospice New Zealand: www.hospice.org.nz
Lewy Body Dementia Association: www.lewybodydementia.org

Movement Disorder Society (MDS): www.movementdisorders.org
National Institute of Neurological Disorders and Stroke (US):
    www.ninds.nih.gov/disorders/disorder_index.htm
National Institutes of Health (US): www.nih.gov
National Institutes of Health – National Institute on Aging (US):
    www.nia.nih.gov
Oz Care Dementia Support: www.dementiasupport.com.au
Parkinson's Australia: www.parkinsons.org.au
Parkinson's New Zealand: www.parkinsons.org.nz
Parkinson's UK: www.parkinsons.org.uk
Parkinsons USA: www.apdaparkinson.org
Patient.co.uk: www.patient.co.uk
WEKA (What Everybody Keeps Asking, disability information):
    www.weka.net.nz
World Health Organization: www.who.int

For people with early-stage dementia who are computer-literate
Alzheimer's Association (US): www.alz.org/living_with_alzheimers_4521.asp
Alzheimer's Australia: www.fightdementia.org.au/understanding-
    dementia/section-8-about-you-information-for-people-with-
    dementia.aspx
Alzheimer Society Canada: www.alzheimer.ca/en/Living-with-dementia/
    I-have-dementia
Dementia Advocacy and Support Network International: www.
    dasninternational.org

Information about the brain
Centre for Brain Research, University of Auckland: www.fmhs.auckland.
    ac.nz/faculty/cbr
Neurological Foundation of New Zealand: www.neurological.org.nz

Financial planning and budgeting
Australia: MoneySmart, www.moneysmart.gov.au
New Zealand: Sorted, www.sorted.org.nz

Select Bibliography

Books

Archibald, Carole and Charlie Murphy (eds), *Activities and People with Dementia Involving Family Carers*, Dementia Services Development Centre, Activities Series, University of Stirling, 1999

Bell, Virginia and David Troxel, *The Best Friends Approach to Alzheimer's Care*, MacLennan & Petty, 1997

Boden (aka Bryden), Christine, *Who Will I Be When I Die?* HarperCollins Religious, 1998

Boss, Pauline: *Loving Someone Who Has Dementia: How to Find Hope while Coping with Stress and Grief*, Jossey-Bass, 2011

Brocx, Suzanne, et al., *A Guide for Carers: A Booklet for Those whose Loved Ones Are Living with Terminal Illness* (adapted from *A Guide for Caregivers*, GlaxoSmithKline Canada), Hospice New Zealand, 2004

Brotchie, Jane, *Caring for Someone with Dementia*, Age Concern Books, 2003

Cayton, Harry, Nori Graham and James Warner, *Dementia: Alzheimer's and Other Dementias at Your Fingertips*, 2nd edn, Class Publishing, 2002

Clark, Alison, Jackie Holland and Jef Smith, *Windows to a Damaged World: Advice and Help for Older People*, Alzheimer's Disease Society UK, 1996

Connor, Jim, *A Funny Thing Happened on the Way to the Nursing Home: A Different Handbook for Carers of Dementia Patients*, BookBound Publishing, 1997

Select Bibliography

Copeman-High, Barbara, *Elsie's Silent Cries: A True Life Experience Coping with Alzheimer's*, FP Comrie Publications, 2000

Crisp, Jane, *Keeping in Touch with Someone Who Has Alzheimer's*, Ausmed Publications, 2000

Gillies, Andrea, *Keeper: Living with Nancy: A Journey into Alzheimer's*, Short Books, 2009

Graboys, Thomas with Peter Zheutlin, *Life in the Balance: A Physician's Memoir of Life, Love, and Loss with Parkinson's Disease and Dementia*, Sterling Publishing, 2008

Irving, Tricia, *Rain, Hail or Shine: Exploring Change, Loss and Grief in a Carer's World*, Skylight, 2005

Jenkins, Deirdre AL, *Intimate Caring Skills: Urinary and Faecal Incontinence, A Heightened Problem when Dementia is a Factor*, University of Stirling, 1999

Knocker, Sally, *The Alzheimer's Society Book of Activities*, Alzheimer's Society UK, 2002

Kübler-Ross, Elisabeth, *On Death and Dying*, Macmillan, 1969

Kübler-Ross, Elisabeth and David Kessler, *Life Lessons*, Simon & Schuster/Touchstone, 2002

Kuhn, Daniel, *Alzheimer's Early Stages: First Steps in Caring and Treatment*, Hunter House, 1999

Lieberman, Abraham, and Frank Williams, *Parkinson's Disease: The Complete Guide for Patients and Caregivers*, Simon & Schuster, 1993

McCarthy, Bernie, *Hearing the Person with Dementia: Person-centred Approaches to Communication for Families and Caregivers*, Jessica Kingsley, 2011

MacKinlay, Elizabeth and Corrine Trevitt, *Facilitating Spiritual Reminiscence for Older People with Dementia: A Learning Package*, Centre for Ageing and Pastoral Studies, 2006

Mace, Nancy L and Peter V Rabins, *The 36-Hour Day: A Family Guide to Caring for People Who Have Alzheimer Disease, Related Dementias, and Memory Loss*, 5th ed., Johns Hopkins University Press, 2011

Marshall, Mary (ed.), *Working with Dementia: Guidelines for Professionals*, Venture Press, 1990

Millen, Julia, *Dilemma of Dementia*, Lansdowne Press, 1985
Mooney, Sharon Fish, *Alzheimer's: Caring for Your Loved One, Caring for Yourself*, Lion Book, 2008
Morrish, Kate, *Do I Like the Taste of That? Caring for a Loved One with Alzheimer's*, Flip Publishing, 1999
Ognowska-Coates, Halina, *I'm Still Elva Inside*, Bridget Williams Books, 1993
—— *Remember Me: Photographs and Stories of Living with Dementia/Alzheimer's Disease*, Alzheimers New Zealand, 2002
Perkins, Chris, *Dementia: A New Zealand Guide*, 2nd edn, Random House, 2006
Powell, Jenny, *Care to Communicate: Helping the Older Person with Dementia, A Practical Guide for Care Workers*, Hawker Publishers, 2000
Raushi, Thaddeus, *A View From Within: Living with Early-onset Alzheimer's*, Northeastern New York Chapter Alzheimer's Disease and Related Disorders Association, 2001
Robinson, Anne, Beth Spencer and Laurie White, *Understanding Difficult Behaviors: Some Practical Suggestions for Coping with Alzheimer's Disease and Related Illnesses*, Geriatric Education Center of Michigan, 1996
Rubinstein, Nataly, *Alzheimer's Disease and Other Dementias: The Caregiver's Complete Survival Guide*, Two Harbors Press, 2011
Sachs, Oliver, *Musicophilia*, Alfred A Knopf, 2007
Sargeant, Delys and Anne Unkenstein, *Remembering Well: How Memory Works and What to Do When It Doesn't*, Allen & Unwin, 1998
Schnarch, David, *Passionate Marriage*, Henry Holt, 1997
Sharma, Nutan and Elaine Richman, *Parkinson's Disease and the Family*, Harvard University Press, 2005
Simpson, Joe, *Touching the Void*, Vintage Books, 2004
Talbot, Marianne, *Keeping Mum: Caring for Someone with Dementia*, Hay House, 2011
Wayman, Laura, *A Loving Approach to Dementia Care: Making Meaningful Connections with the Person Who Has Alzheimer's Disease and Other Dementia or Memory Loss*, Johns Hopkins University Press, 2011

Whitworth, Helen Buell and James Whitworth, *Lewy Body Dementia: A Caregivers' Guide*, Demos Health, 2011

Wilson, Andrew Norman, *Iris As I Knew Her*, Hutchinson, 2003

Zeisel, John, *I'm Still Here: A Breakthrough Approach to Understanding Someone Living with Alzheimer's*, Piatkus, 2010

Articles, booklets, pamphlets and papers

'The Dementia Booklet: Information for Carers, Family and Whanau Following a Diagnosis of Dementia', Alzheimers New Zealand, 2008

'Everyday People and Mental Illness', New Zealand Ministry of Health/ Manatu Hauora

Ferman, Tanis J, Glenn Smith and Briana Melom, 'Understanding Behavioral Changes in Dementia', available online at: www.lbda.org/node/203

'A Guide for Carers: A Booklet for Those Whose Loved Ones Are Living with a Terminal Illness', Hospice New Zealand, 2008

'Information Kit for the Over 60s', Jim Anderton's Electorate Office, New Zealand

McNaughton, Brian, 'God in Dementia' *Alzheimer's News New Zealand*. Issue 50, June 2002

'Mental Health Services for Older People', Auckland District Health Board/Te Toka Tumai, April 2008

'Residential Care for People with Dementia: Information for People with Dementia, Their Carers and Families', Alzheimers New Zealand, 2006

Snow, Barry and Lorraine Macdonald, *Parkinson's Disease*, Parkinson's New Zealand, 2000

Whorwood, Delyse, *A Caregiver's Guide to Looking after a Person with Progressive Supranuclear Palsy Syndrome: From a Carer's Viewpoint*, Parkinson's Society of New Zealand, 2005

'Your Brain at Work: Making the Science of Cognitive Fitness Work for You', The Conference Board, and The Dana Alliance for Brain Initiatives, 2008

Newsletters

Headlines, Neurological Foundation of New Zealand national newsletters, 1998–2010
MIND Matters, Alzheimers Auckland, 2004–2012
The Parkinsonian, New Zealand Parkinson's Society, 1994–2010
Penstrokes, Stroke Foundation Northern Region New Zealand, 2004–2012
Positive Directions, Parkinson's Auckland, 1994–2010

DVD

A Thousand Tomorrows – Intimacy, sexuality and Alzheimer's, Educational Media Australia, Nbr: 9-84747 F-1 #54.

Index

abnormal memory loss 24
abuse 306–7
acceptance 27, 57, 76, 79, 113, 272
accountants 59, 63, 64, 200, 285
acetylcholine neurotransmitter 38
acetylcholinesterase enzyme inhibitors *see* anticholinesterases
activities *see* entertainment activities
acupuncture 180–1
adapting the home environment 90–100
advance care planning 64; *see also* long-term care
Age Concern 59
aggression 25–6, 41, 45, 170, 237, 259, 266, 268–79
agitation 79, 105, 107, 132, 151, 161, 170, 178–9, 182, 297
alcohol 30, 49, 105, 112, 178, 208, 227, 230–1, 254, 287
allowances *see* benefits, government; disability allowances
alternative therapies *see* natural therapies

Alzheimer's disease 39–41
  diagnostic guidelines 29
  medical treatments 169
anger 29, 41, 78, 113, 134, 139, 165, 192, 272, 275, 276, 303
anticholinesterases (AChEI) 45, 89, 169–70, 173
antipsychotic drugs 170, 291
antisocial behaviour 47, 107–9
apathy 42, 141, 169
aphasia 138
arguments 104, 148, 262, 296, 304
Aricept 169, 173, 174
armchair activities 202
aromatherapy 181
art activities 197, 203–4
assessment of needs 87–8, 90, 232, 244
assets *see* legal and money matters
axons 37, 38

ball games 191–2
bathrooms 94–6, 218–19, 234, 236

baths and bathing 94–5, 106, 165, 181, 208, 219, 232, 233, 234–7
becoming a carer *see* caregivers
bedsores 98, 99, 238, 242, 288
bed-wetting 247–9
benefits, government 62, 63, 64, 169, 285, 312–13; *see also* community funding; disability allowances
bladder 180, 182, 248–9, 254, 288
blood pressure 41, 82, 132, 136, 170, 176, 311
boredom 151, 256
bowel accidents 182, 250, 252–5
brain banks 313
brain functions 36–8
brain research centres 321

card games 197
caregivers 69–80, 111–16, 135, 270
Carer's Code 72, 113–14
carers' education programme 135
catastrophic reactions 274–6
catheters 248–9
celebrating festivals and gifts 207–8
choking emergencies 228
Citizens Advice Bureau 59, 72
cleaning 94, 199, 249–50, 252–3
clothing 19, 206, 208, 213, 216, 224, 238–43, 245, 258, 295–6; *see also* showering and dressing
cognitive decline 24, 27, 30

medical treatments 170
communication 140–54; *see also* non-verbal communication; speech and language difficulties
asking questions and resolving problems 78–9, 290
covering up or denial 50–1
keeping in touch 305
reluctance to accept diagnosis 50
reminding and recording details 73–5
sex and feelings 159–60
talking and planning together 51–2
telling employers 57–8
telling family members 52–5
telling friends and colleagues 55–7
with needs assessors 87
community funding 90; *see also* government funding
complementary therapies *see* natural therapies
confusion 23–4, 26–7, 35–6, 40, 41, 63, 105, 170, 227, 259, 291
constipation 227, 253–4, 291
continence pads 247–8
contracts
resolving home caregiving issues 78–9, 158
with care facilities 293, 308
cooking and baking activities 197–8

counsellors and counselling 66, 72, 99, 131, 162, 317
court orders 63

dance activities 199–200
day and respite care 88
dealing with health professionals 29–33, 81–9, 85–7
dealing with the diagnosis 50–8
death 26, 38, 41, 310–19; *see also* final days; legal and money matters
death grip 276–7
dehydration 177–8, 227, 255, 270; *see also* drinking
delirium 170, 266–7; *see also* fevers; hallucinations and misinterpretations; paranoia
delusions *see* hallucinations and misinterpretations
dendrites 36, 38
denial 51
dentist 120
dentures 142
depression 29, 30, 105, 131–2, 156, 181, 278
  in caregivers 113, 131–2, 135
diagnosis 29–34, 39, 85–6, 137, 197
Diagnostic Guidelines for Alzheimer's Disease (US) 29
difficult behaviours 101–9
disability allowances 169, 247; *see also* benefits, government; community funding

distance caring 112
doctors and specialists, *see* dealing with health professionals
Donezil *see* Aricept
dressing *see* showering and dressing
dressmaking or fashion activities 198
drinking 153, 223–31; *see also* dehydration
driving 54–5, 123–5
drowsiness or sleeplessness *see* tiredness
drugs *see* medications
dyskinesia (involuntary movements) 172
dysthymia (mild depression) 132

early-onset dementia 49
early signs 23–8
eating and drinking *see* food and drink; drinking
eating out 223, 231
echoing 147; *see also* repetition
emergency situations 75, 175
  choking emergencies 228
  useful phone numbers, notes, instructions 92, 175
emotions 19, 113, 127–39, 159–61, 204, 268–79, 302–5, 313–15
employers 57–8
encouragement by participation 195–6
enduring powers of attorney (EPOA) 60–5, 153–4

entertainment activities 194–209, 299
enzymes 38, 169
estates and trusts 62–6
Exelon 119, 169
exercises and physical activities 87, 182–93, 200

falls 46, 94, 177
family and friends 50–66, 71, 81, 85, 87, 92, 99, 110–16, 135, 146, 164, 205, 207–8; *see also* support groups
fantasies 101–3
feelings *see* emotions
fevers 170, 176, 227, 270; *see also* delirium
final days 310–19; *see also* death
finances *see* legal and money matters
fishing activities 198
following behaviour 80
food and drink 223–31
foreplay *see* sexual relations
forgetfulness 23–4, 49, 262–3
forms of dementia 39–49
friends *see* family and friends
fronto-temporal dementias (FTD) 46–8, 271
frustration 41, 75, 134–5, 182, 268–9
full-time care 64, 283–309; *see also* long-term care
funeral planning 311–12

gardening activities 152, 198–9, 201, 212, 287–8
geriatrician *see* specialists
gifts 208
goals 51–2, 113–14, 179
golfing activities 191, 199
government funding *see* benefits, government
grief 309, 313–18

hair care 237–8
hallucinations and misinterpretations 25, 45, 96, 132, 170, 263–6, 270, 308; *see also* delirium; paranoia
handrails, ramps and safety gates 90–1, 95–6
headaches 112, 132, 176
hearing aids 141–2
hearing loss 141–2, 144, 176, 197, 270, 278
Heimlich manoeuvre 228
help in the home 87, 233
herbalism 180
holidays and travel 210–20
home care activities 199
homeopathy 180
hospital care 308–9
humour 136–7, 153, 263, 274; *see also* laughter
Huntington's disease 48–9

'I' messages 71, 132–4, 272, 306
impatience 19, 134, 255

Index   331

impulse control disorders 171
incontinence 240, 244–55, 288, 291
independence and safety 119–26
infections 132, 178, 180, 227 266, 270–1, 308
inside activities 201–2
instructions, giving 144–6, 237, 269
insurances 63, 64, 86, 125, 215
intercourse *see* sexual relations
internet 59, 72
intimacy, love and sex 44, 51, 155–66
investments 63; *see also* legal and money matters
involuntary grip 276–7
involuntary movements (dyskinesia) 172
irritability 131, 132

joint bank accounts 62
joint ownership 63
journal keeping 18, 75–6, 83–4, 135, 160, 254, 278

language *see* speech and language difficulties
laughter 18, 111, 136–7, 141, 144, 145, 153, 163, 184, 219, 233, 255, 272, 276, 289; *see also* humour
legal and money matters 59–66, 122–3, 312–13, 321; *see also* investments
legal professionals 59–65

Lewy body dementia (LBD) 38, 44–6, 89, 90, 169, 170, 184, 186
life books 74, 105, 203
listening skills 111, 133, 135, 141, 143, 151, 298, 309
living wills 64; *see also* wills
loneliness 115, 130–1, 162, 165, 256, 289, 303
long-term care 63–4, 283–309; *see also* advance care planning; full-time care
love *see* intimacy, love and sex
lying or making things up 101–2

Madopar 170, 174
malnutrition 305
mask-like features 105, 149
massage 87, 180, 228
medical breakthroughs 171
medical folders 74–5, 84, 88, 172, 175, 289
medications 169–81; *see also* drugs; natural therapies
  and alcohol 105, 229, 230
  and day and respite care 88
  disposal of unwanted medications 89
  and facility policy 291
  incompatibilities and side-effects 45, 46, 129, 132, 142, 162, 171–3, 180, 227, 238, 243, 254, 267, 268, 270, 278
  managing medications 89, 91, 174–6, 285

new prescriptions 172–4
over-medicating 172
over-the-counter products 75, 171
reviewing medications 173
safekeeping and dispensing 175–6
travel arrangements 214
memory
Alzheimer's disease 39–40
Huntington's disease 48
Lewy body dementia 45
losing things, forgetfulness 23–4, 276
and memories 204
natural remedies 171
Parkinson's disease dementia 46
reminding and recording 73, 135, 157–8
strokes 42–4
travel arrangements 214–15
memory clinics 86
mental health authority 85–6, 169
mini mental status examination (MMSE) 30, 173
misinterpretations *see* hallucinations and misinterpretations
mobility aids 90, 95–6, 98–9, 187–8, 190, 205, 212, 214, 215, 233, 245, 290
mobility assessments 87
mobility concession cards 123
modesty 232–3, 239
money matters *see* legal and money matters

mood swings 29, 35, 105–7, 112, 150, 182, 228
motivation 42, 183, 196
music and dance 40, 43–4, 106, 138, 188, 195, 199–200, 205, 208, 228, 275

nail care 237
natural therapies 179–81
needs assessors and coordinators 87–8, 90, 232, 244
nerves 36
neurologists *see* specialists
neurotransmitters 38, 44, 169
NICE Guideline on Dementia (UK) 29
night lights 208, 287, 294
non-verbal communication 111, 145, 149, 151, 153, 272
normal memory loss 23, 24
nutritional therapy 180, 229

occupational therapists 87, 90, 92, 95, 96, 97, 187, 224, 244, 245, 246, 289
office work activities 200
organ donations 313
organisations and support groups 114–16, 169, 320–1
outings 73, 144, 205–6, 288, 302; *see also* visiting
overseas travel *see* travelling arrangements
over-the-counter medications 75

paranoia 262–63; *see also* delirium; hallucinations and misinterpretations
paraphrasing 143
Parkinson's disease 31–3, 38, 44–5, 46, 320–1
and Lewy body dementia 44–5
Parkinson's disease dementia (PDD) 46, 90, 92, 123, 131, 137, 160, 165, 170, 173, 174, 184, 185, 223, 227, 229, 251, 253, 271, 320–1
personal grooming 237–8; *see also* showering and dressing
pets 155, 203, 299
pharmacists 88–9, 99, 171, 175–6, 227, 247
photos 74, 76, 102, 112, 202–3, 207, 208, 256, 258, 287, 294, 316
physical activities 106, 163, 178–9, 182–93; *see also* entertainment
physical contact 152, 269, 305, 315
physical examination 29, 141
physiotherapists *see* specialists
Pick's disease 47
pill dispensers 175
police 53, 99, 258, 260
polypharmacy 172
power of attorney *see* enduring power of attorney
precautions *see* safety precautions

prescriptions 82, 88, 89, 142, 172, 214, 217, 229, 239, 285
privacy laws 85, 162
problem-solving 36, 72, 133, 279
prognosis 38
psychogeriatricians *see* specialists
psychotherapy 179

questions to ask
  facility managers 286–7
  health professionals 30–1, 81, 84–7, 172, 174
  legal professionals 64
  support groups 114–15

radio and television programmes 101, 106, 199, 201, 208, 269, 274, 298
reading glasses 142, 278
reassessment 308
recordkeeping *see* journal keeping
recuperation for carers 116
reflexology 179
regular activities and routines *see* routines
religion or spirituality 137–9
relocation 308
Reminyl 169
repetition 77, 147; *see also* echoing
resources 320–1
respect 39, 81, 87, 155–6, 233, 298
respite care 88, 111, 114–15, 149, 240, 242, 286

restraints 170, 290–1
ropinirole 46, 171
routines 47, 72–3, 77, 80, 106, 144, 182–3, 193, 195, 206, 219, 235, 238–9, 256, 270, 279, 287, 294, 296, 298–9

safety precautions 90–100, 119–26, 174, 219, 257–9, 265, 275
secure facilities 200, 261, 286–7
sedatives 105, 170, 184, 291
self-care 112–14, 116; see also support groups
sense of humour see humour
sexual behaviour in public see antisocial behaviour
sexual relations 155–66; see also intimacy, love and sex
shaving 236, 238
short-term memory loss 39, 42, 45, 60
showering and dressing 72, 78–9, 94–6, 145, 165, 208, 212, 215, 218–19, 232–43, 245, 288, 306–7; see also clothing; personal grooming
signals 143, 148–51, 250, 257
Sinemet 170, 174
sleeping 45, 96–7, 98, 106, 112, 132, 155, 170, 172, 178–9, 182, 184, 240, 269, 291, 303, 315
social life 71, 130–1, 166, 171, 207–8, 287, 304

Specialised Early Care for Alzheimer's (SPECAL) 77
specialists 29, 31, 33, 85–7, 181, 283, 289, 308
speech and language difficulties 41–3, 48, 138, 142, 145–54, 227, 246, 266, 286, 305; see also communication; non-verbal communication
spirituality 137–9
stiffness 44–6, 77, 170, 240
strokes 41–4, 49, 176–7, 310, 311, 320–1; see also transient ischaemic attacks (TIAs); vascular dementia
  and communication 148–9
  epilepsy 44
  exercises 190
  left-hemisphere damage 43
  right-hemisphere damage 43–4
suicidal thoughts 112
sundowning/twilighting 105–6, 182, 208, 271, 278
support groups 15, 89, 114–15, 131, 135, 162, 194, 210, 247, 255, 260, 286, 292, 304, 316; see also family and friends; self-care
supra-pubic catheter 248–9
swallowing 40, 48, 226–8, 305, 311
symptoms 16, 23–32, 52, 56, 72, 81, 84, 85, 110, 184, 262, 266, 275
  Alzheimer's disease 39
  dehydration 177–8, 227